Engaging a Community of Hope

Engaging *a* Community *of* Hope

Empowering Collegiate Leaders for Student Recovery

CO-AUTHORED BY

Kelsey L. Austin-Wright, MS, LMFT
AND Nathan R. Patzke, MDIV

FOREWORD BY
DR. Austin McNeill Brown, MSW, PHD

CASCADE *Books* • Eugene, Oregon

Cascade Books
An Imprint of Wipf and Stock Publishers
199 W. 8th Ave., Suite 3
Eugene, OR 97401

www.wipfandstock.com

PAPERBACK ISBN: 978-1-6667-8249-3
HARDCOVER ISBN: 978-1-6667-8250-9
EBOOK ISBN: 978-1-6667-8251-6

Cataloguing-in-Publication data:

Names: Austin-Wright, Kelsey L., author. | Patzke, Nathan R., author. | Brown, Austin McNeill, foreword.

Title: Engaging a community of hope : empowering collegiate leaders for student recovery / by Kelsey L. Austin-Wright and Nathan R. Patzke ; foreword by Austin McNeill Brown.

Description: Eugene, OR: Cascade Books, 2025 | Includes bibliographical references.

Identifiers: ISBN 978-1-6667-8249-3 (paperback) | ISBN 978-1-6667-8250-9 (hardcover) | ISBN 978-1-6667-8251-6 (ebook)

Subjects: LCSH: Drug addiction. | Alcoholism. | Drug addiction—Treatment—young adults.

Classification: HV5801 E3935 2025 (paperback) | HV5801 (ebook)

VERSION NUMBER 04/25/25

Permission, for print and online usage, for the list of known CRPs in Appendix 1 was obtained by ARHE.

To our students at the Beauchamp Addiction Recovery Center. Past. Present. Future. We truly would not be where we are without each and every one of you.

With Love,

Kelsey and Nathan

Contents

Foreword

TALK TO ANY CURRENT or former student associated with Collegiate Recovery Programs (CRPs) about their experience, and they will light up instantly and enthusiastically. They will express a deep sense of gratitude and loyalty and cite lifelong friends and colleagues they have made through their collegiate recovery experience. CRPs throughout the country have given thousands of students a chance at a college education that, for many, had seemed out of reach. Without a CRP, I personally would not have been eligible to attend my alma mater due to the wreckage of my multiple academic failures pursuant to my addictions. Today, thanks to CRPs, there are thousands of professionals, scientists, and scholars who could say the same.

Addiction and successful college education, for whatever reasons, often act in contradiction for those who develop these disorders. Heavy drug and alcohol use is often antithetical to academic achievement in college. Nevertheless, the critical hope that collegiate recovery provides is that recovery from addiction seems to work concomitantly with higher education, unlocking the academic potential of those in recovery who often have unique potentials and hidden capacities. The performance of students in recovery speaks for itself. Collegiate recovery students continually exceed institutional and national grade point averages, they graduate at a higher rate, and from year to year, they move along in their education either at a faster or expected pace, graduating on time and with excellent grades. Recovery and education work synergistically; the social capital gained with a four-year degree stabilizes long-term recovery, and the values and principles of recovery bolster the student's positive attitudes, academic discipline, and willingness to put forth the effort to succeed at high academic levels above and beyond their non-recovering peers. In many ways, the marriage of recovery and higher education through CRPs creates an ideal symbiosis that results in high levels of academic success and long-term stability for recovery from addiction.

A four-year degree is a significant investment in today's competitive and often expensive collegiate environment. The statistics on health determinants, well-being, chronic diseases, and overall mental health for non-college-educated populations are poor and declining across all measures.[1] Thus, in the United States today, there is often little choice for accessing and maintaining a middle-class lifestyle without higher education. A college degree is vital to living with a modicum of stability, wellness, and security in America today. The stakes are indeed high. Collegiate recovery opens up new terrain for those who have struggled with education and addiction, and in doing so, collegiate recovery serves an integral and often invisible population on today's college campuses. Opening doors and ensuring success are what recovery programs are all about.

This concise manual offers a succinct and transparent resource to those who operate CRPs or those looking to develop a program like this on their own campus. It may also be helpful for those seeking to learn about or understand CRPs, whom they serve, and how they operate at the institutional and community level. In sum, this manual should be on the bookshelf of most college administrators, CRP managers, and researchers seeking to understand the mutually beneficial relationship between recovery from substance use disorder and these academically based support programs that seek to meet their unique needs within the campus environment.

—Dr. Austin McNeill Brown, MSW, PhD

---

1. Case and Deaton, "Great Divide," 17.

Acknowledgments

MANY HAVE IMPACTED THE development of my (Kelsey's) character, my pursuit of knowledge, and my career. To everyone, I am grateful. While I cannot pinpoint an exact time in my life that I decidedly embraced the creation of belonging, advocacy, and support as a calling, I can certainly identify a few contributors that enabled my trajectory.

To my husband, thank you for your patience, and for understanding from the very beginning of our relationship that I will forever keep myself busy learning and sharing that knowledge with others. Thank you for supporting me through late nights and early mornings of research and writing. Your encouragement, and pride in me, mean the world and more.

To my parents, thank you for instilling in me the desire to learn. Your efforts to be present for every school function and extracurricular event can still be felt as I continue to learn and grow. I can feel your support even from afar, and it is one of my greatest joys to make you both proud.

To the Center for Young Adult Addiction and Recovery at Kennesaw State University, thank you. Thank you for introducing me to the field of collegiate recovery, and for embracing me as a young recovery ally. Thank you for giving me a platform for education and advocacy as a peer health educator and as an undergraduate research assistant. To Austin Brown, I am incredibly grateful for your presence at KSU and for your mentorship of the inexperienced, eager researcher in me. Your recommendation to attend Texas Tech University and study marriage and family therapy has developed into a career I never knew I could love so much. Thanks for believing in me.

In contemplation of those who have made my (Nathan's) life more enriched and learned, I have difficulty naming specific people or places that have given me the privileges that I hold today.

My parents laid the foundation of what it means to work hard, and to value human lives regardless of various factors. I thank my parents, as well as my two sisters, for instilling in me the desire to treat others with respect, love, and charity.

To my wife, Callie, who, on countless occasions, has gone to be alone so that I may stay up to research, write, or rest. You are the source of my drive and integrity. I cannot express to you the ways in which I feel about you in mere words.

To my closest friends who have continuously supported and encouraged me, and who have helped in maintaining my mental, physical, and spiritual health. People like Rev. Hannah Brown and her spouse, Jesse Pipes, are two named friends who provided me with feedback and general rest throughout the entire process of writing this book. Thank you, my friends.

Lastly to Kelsey, my co-author. Not only are you my supervisor at Baylor's CRP, but you are also a consistent source of positive energy throughout my week. The short time period, which admittedly we alone were responsible for, made writing more stressful than usual for me. It was your constant mental support that allowed me to finish my researching, writing, and editing for this book. I am very grateful.

The two of us have much to be thankful for during the completion of this project. In partnership, there are certain individuals whom we'd like to acknowledge prior to the start of this book.

To Rev. Dr. Erin Moniz and Dr. Gaynor Yancey, we are truly appreciative. You two helped to review our manuscript and assess its voice, integrity, and vocabulary. Without the knowledge and experiences you two hold, this book would not be where it is today. We cannot express our gratitude enough in the short space we have here.

To all of our endorsers, we extend our utmost and sincere thanks. Your effort in showcasing our book means more to us than you know. It is with your help that this book is as complete as it is now. We cannot thank you enough.

For Dr. Austin Brown we are certainly appreciative. Dr. Brown has not only invested in Kelsey personally and professionally but has also provided a Foreword for this book. In this Foreword, Dr. Brown showcases the necessity for appropriate collegiate recovery, and its results when done in an educational context. Dr. Brown, we thank you for your gift of scholarship and writing ability.

Lastly, but certainly of no less importance, we'd like to mention our place of employment, Baylor University's Beauchamp Addiction Recovery Center. This place is more than a workplace, it is a place in which we are inspired, educated, and welcomed. It is a place in which we feel that we can be our complete, genuine selves. It is also a place that shows the two of us the most grace. To every student, past and present; to every donor; to every person in higher administration, we thank you. We love this place for what it is: a place of rest for the restless, a place of peace for the peaceless, and a home for the homeless. Without the BARC, this book would not exist. We are grateful.

Introduction

What Are CRPs?

Collegiate Recovery Programs (CRPs), also known as Collegiate Recovery Communities (CRCs), exist on college campuses to provide support, advocacy, and resources for students in recovery. They support students' academic success, emotional growth, and sustained recovery. The first CRP started at Brown University in 1977. There are now over 150 programs that vary widely to meet each institution's unique needs.[1] These programs provide accountability and safe spaces for individuals navigating the nuances of higher education while in recovery.

The program started at Texas Tech University (TTU) in 1986 proved to be very helpful for students and now serves as a model for collegiate recovery. TTU then received a Replication Grant in 2005 that allowed them to help other universities across the nation create CRPs. This led to a collegiate recovery boom across the nation as universities gained the knowledge and confidence to establish their own programs to meet the needs of their students in recovery. As more programs developed at various institutions, a need for community, shared knowledge, and programming growth arose. TTU met this need by hosting the

1. Pennelle, "History of Collegiate Recovery," para. 3.

first national collegiate recovery conference in 2010. The Association for Recovery in Higher Education (ARHE) was formed at the conference and incorporated in 2011.

CRPs serve their role in addressing the public health concern of young adult substance use. The prevalence of alcohol and other drug use on college campuses can serve as a threat to sobriety. CRPs have provided the structure and support needed for students in recovery to navigate college experiences and academic pressures without jeopardizing their recovery gains.

Colleges and universities serve diverse demographics of students, and each campus develops its own unique culture. For this reason, no two CRPs are quite the same. For a CRP to be successful, it must create a sanctuary as well as a sense of belonging for the students of a particular institution. Some programs may be more structured to provide an added layer of accountability for students seeking academic success at a competitive university, while others may be more open and focused on a sense of belonging on a campus that carries stigma towards individuals in recovery.

It is not uncommon for programs to utilize an application system to filter students that may participate in CRCs. Some programs choose to uphold students to membership requirements such as minimum sobriety time, minimum GPA, the expected number of peer support meetings attended each week, and other factors. This approach is especially useful for programs that offer scholarships for students in recovery, facilitate research in their CRP, and offer recovery housing.

Other colleges and universities take more of an "open door" approach to collegiate recovery. They may share a space with the Wellness Department or prevention specialists, and they may want to include more allies in their community. This setup can be especially helpful for institutions that have an underlying stigma of "otherness" for individuals who struggle with substance use disorders (SUDs) and other behavioral addictions. Creating a safe space on campus that is welcoming to any student, in recovery or not, allows space for allies and sober-curious students to also utilize the CRP.

Despite the differences in programming, all CRPs share a common goal: to provide student support in higher education. Students' needs shift over the years, and CRPs must be intentional about attuning to cultural trends in higher education and their own institution's gaps in student support. The ARHE provides community, education, and resources for the growing number of professionals, allies, and students in the collegiate recovery field to better support recovering students in unique ways.

While there is a lack of existing research on the benefits of collegiate recovery as a field, individual CRPs have shared their own independent studies demonstrating the efficacy of their programs. TTU's CRP found that their students maintained a higher GPA and had a higher graduation rate than the general TTU student population.[2] Being engaged in a CRP can provide the necessary support for recovering students to excel in higher education—an opportunity that may not have otherwise been possible for them.

Difference(s) Between Treatment and Collegiate Recovery

The treatment of addiction is often conceptualized as a continuum of care. Collegiate recovery is not generally included as part of formalized treatment for SUDs or other process addictions. Rather, CRPs are utilized as ongoing support further down the continuum to help sustain long-term recovery. Not all students involved in CRPs will have completed a treatment program. Completion of treatment is not a necessary requirement for most CRPs, but it is important to note that CRPs should not be utilized as a substitute for treatment.

The severity of symptoms and dysfunction caused by a SUD or other process addiction are the determining factors for placing individuals in the appropriate level of care. A student experiencing a severe SUD with significant consequences on their mental, physical, or relational wellness should be recommended to a higher

---

2. Harris et al., "Achieving Systems-Based Sustained Recovery," 234.

level of care such as residential treatment or an intensive outpatient program (IOP). These higher levels of care are intervention-driven and facilitated by licensed clinicians.

Once a student has reached a level of stability and is no longer struggling with compulsive use, he or she may be a good fit for the support of a CRP. CRPs are peer-driven, and provide students continued care through peer-support meetings, individual support from CRP staff, and sometimes substance-free recovery housing. This level of care is most appropriate for individuals experiencing lower severity symptoms of a SUD or process addiction or who have sustained recovery time already and are looking for a supportive community.

Mental Health Support on College Campuses

In the fall of 2021, over 50 percent of college students reported moderate psychological distress and an additional 22 percent reported severe psychological distress.[3] Academic pressure, social isolation, financial insecurity, time management, sense of self, and other stressors can impact the mental well-being of students. Navigating these stressors on top of recovery from SUDs can be especially challenging.

College campuses not only support students' academic success but also often support individuals' mental well-being. Many departments within an institution may work together to address students' mental health needs. Wellness departments, counseling centers, CRPs, spiritual life, and other offices often pool resources to meet the growing demand from students. The Association of University and College Counseling Center Directors reported that during the 2021–2022 school year, 85.5 percent of college counseling centers reported an increase in utilization of their services.[4]

3. American College Health Association, "Executive Summary Fall 2021," 12.

4. Association for University and College Counseling Center Directors, "Annual Survey 2021," 6.

More students are taking advantage of the mental health resources offered on campuses each year.

CRPs, while not always clinical in nature, offer support for the well-being of students by strengthening recovery capital, offering peer support, and providing mental health resources. Recovery and mental health overlap significantly, and CRPs can fill a gap that counseling centers or wellness departments sometimes miss. As the demand for mental health services increases, so too will the need for CRPs.

The Shifting Language Around Addiction/Recovery

The language in the addiction recovery field is ever evolving. The field has historically used terms such as "addict" and "alcoholic" to describe individuals experiencing SUDs. These labels diminished the multifaceted nature of humans and minimized the positive aspects of individuals. It was also common to refer to drug tests as "dirty" when failed, and "clean" when passed. This language attached morality to SUDs, further stigmatizing the individuals who were experiencing them. It was not uncommon to hear descriptions such as "hopeless," "hostile," and "manipulative" assigned to individuals diagnosed with SUDs. Negative descriptors such as these reinforced the choice model of addiction and continued to marginalize individuals with SUDs.

The culture has shifted positively to be more strengths-based and destigmatizing. While individuals may choose to identify however they would like, and some programs use specific terms to describe themselves, the field has shifted to more person-first language. For example, some individuals self-identify as "addicts" or "alcoholics." This identity should be respected. This book, as well as many CRPs, will use the terminology "individuals with SUDs" to be person-first.

The field of collegiate recovery strives to recognize ways in which students self-advocate and utilize services and support. Rather than referring to students as "lazy" or "resistant," CRP professionals realize that students may be ambivalent, working to build hope, or simply not ready. Student "weaknesses" are reframed as barriers to change or unmet needs. Sustaining a healthy and supportive CRC environment requires intentional compassionate language.

The authors of this book are intentional about using language that is recovery-friendly and inclusive while also acknowledging that an individual may resonate with different terminology. In a world of changing semantics, intentionality to humanize and destigmatize the experience of recovery is most important.

How to Use This Resource

This project is one that, we believe, will be helpful to those feeling the desire to assist students in addiction recovery. With this belief comes the logical implication that some readers will approach this resource from diverse backgrounds, scenarios, and access to institutional resources. The information covered in this book will serve recovery allies, higher education professionals, CRP staff, and students in recovery. Parents of CRP students, CRP donors, allied churches, recovery high school staff, and social workers may also find this resource useful.

We hope that this book can be used "as needed," with different chapters on the various aspects of collegiate recovery. Readers can orient themselves to that which they desire to gain from it, rather than needing to read the whole book for merely one implementable resource. Each section may serve as an asset in different seasons of a CRP's development and as student needs shift.

It will be beneficial for readers to consult the table of contents to address their unique experiences and needs. While these chapters contain valuable and insightful information regarding the implementation of CRPs, they are not exhaustive. Throughout our experience in collegiate recovery, we have found that certain issues are resolved on a "trial-and-error" basis. This means that some of the functions found in this book may not work for some programs or initiatives. With that being said, we hope to provide, at the very least, a starting point to a healthy and long-lasting resolution to the issues our readers may find themselves in.

A Note to Our Readers

As you continue throughout our book, or only find yourself in certain necessary sections for specific scenarios, we hope that our resource proves beneficial to collegiate recovery professionals, allies, and students in recovery. We welcome you to approach the contents of this resource with an open mind and with cautious optimism. After all, you have decided through picking this book that your students in recovery need something more. We praise you for that. Whether you find yourself in a cubicle or on the front lines of collegiate recovery, we believe in you. Blessings on you, your employees and volunteers, your institution, and, ultimately, your students.

—————— Chapter 1 ——————

Observations of Collegiate Recovery Throughout the Pandemic Era

As MENTIONED IN THE Introduction, this resource can be used "as needed" in certain scenarios that readers may be facing. This chapter is not necessarily one containing practical advice or guidelines to implement in recovery programs. This chapter will provide some context as to why CRPs are necessary for higher education institutions. The facts and statistics throughout this chapter are just a glimpse into the mind of the college-aged adult and what they face on a daily basis.

In the field of collegiate recovery, it is necessary to discuss the effects of the COVID-19 pandemic on collegiate substance use and misuse. With this preface comes three preconceptions that need to be addressed. First, nothing was immune to the COVID pandemic. Understanding this fact is essential to continue. Second, college-aged students, which for the sake of this book range from eighteen to twenty-five years old, did not benefit from staying home and isolating. Isolation was necessary to prevent the spread of the COVID virus, but that does not mean that the college student was not negatively affected in other ways. Last, college students and the recovery initiatives established for them were negatively affected by the pandemic. It is easy to blame oneself on the lower attendance, higher levels of substance misuse among college students, or the overall rise in hesitation towards addiction recovery that resulted from the pandemic. The goal of this book is to urge CRP professionals not to blame themselves. Collegiate recovery staff must approach this next season by giving themselves grace to continue assisting college students in recovery.

Collegiate Recovery Before the Pandemic

This chapter will first reflect on recovery spaces before the pandemic was made official by the World Health Organization (WHO) in March 2020.[1] The fall semester of 2019 marked a time of tremendous recovery efforts across the nation for not just collegiate leaders, but educational leadership at the K–12 level as well. For example, a nonprofit called the Association of Recovery Schools (ARS) contained at least forty recovery high schools, which are secondary schools with recovery aspects built into the curriculum.[2] These types of initiatives constitute what the recovery industry was like before the pandemic: thriving and innovating. This is not to say that substance use and misuse were not an issue before the pandemic, as around 14.1 percent, or 4.8 million, of the eighteen- to twenty-five-year-olds in the country disclosed SUDs in 2019.[3] This number, as shocking as it may seem, was a decrease from 15.3 percent, or 5.3 million people, in 2015.[4] While the pandemic certainly made these numbers worse, the efforts made by recovery leadership leading up to the pandemic must be acknowledged.

---

1. Centers for Disease Control and Prevention, "COVID-19 Timeline," para. 41.

2. Association of Recovery Schools, "What is a Recovery High School?," para. 1.

3. Han and Piscopo, "2019 National Survey on Drug Use and Health," 41.

4. Han and Piscopo, "2019 National Survey on Drug Use and Health," 41.

It is likely the case that many reading this book who already had institutions of collegiate recovery in place before the pandemic have come to know a direct shift as a result of institutional policies and student isolation. Once bustling recovery spaces on campus now may be sparsely populated. Events that used to be the most popular may lack turnout after students have returned to campus. Rather than thinking of pre-COVID times as the "glory days" of collegiate recovery, this book aims to give readers approaches they can use to rebuild, or start, CRPs at their institution.

Collegiate Recovery During the Pandemic

To speak on recovery initiatives during the pandemic, it is useful to begin with the general restrictions that the pandemic caused in society. First is the limitation of direct human contact. The general six-foot rule that was put into place was to limit the spread of the coronavirus between people. Along with this spacing guideline was the mask mandates that occurred all over the world. Masks were proven to limit the spread and lethality of the virus, coupled with proper distancing between oneself and others.[5]

Although these initiatives from health organizations across the world proved beneficial for the limitation of the spread of the coronavirus, the mental health consequences from such implemented regulations proved to be harmful in hindsight. The collegiate recovery world was forced to shift rapidly, as most others were during the year 2020. Recovery meetings were held online during the first months of the pandemic, as most higher education institutions required all students to finish the semester virtually. As fall 2020 approached, most institutions stayed online, with others requiring heavy masking and social distancing regulations.[6] Instead of the usual back-to-school procedures, collegiate recovery leaders were forced to start innovating, as the health and well-being of their students depended on it.

5. Gandhi et al., "Masks Do More Than Protect," 3063–66.
6. Felson and Adamczyk, "Online or In Person?," 13.

The pandemic did not merely affect collegiate interactions, but also dramatically increased nationwide substance use and misuse. The data from 2019 above did not include the consequences of the pandemic, as it had not been declared a public health emergency by the United States until March 2020.[7] The data from the same survey conducted in 2020 did, however, show the unparalleled effects of the pandemic on substance use and misuse for adults aged eighteen to twenty-five. In 2020 alone, SUDs were disclosed by 24.4 percent, or 8.2 million, of adults in the eighteen- to twenty-five-year age range.[8] This means that in 2020, a quarter of college-aged young adults claimed a substance use disorder. Within the first nine months of America's battle with COVID-19, SUDs rose more than 10 percent in college-aged adults alone.

The results from 2021 only proved the drastic increase in SUDs, and the necessity to shift collegiate recovery even more. In 2021, SUDs appeared in 25.6 percent, or 8.6 million, of adults aged eighteen to twenty-five.[9] More than a full percentage, or about 400,000 more people aged eighteen to twenty-five, disclosed SUDs in 2021. A quarter of all college-aged adults had experienced substance misuse in their life. These lethal statistics provide a glimpse into the shift in substance use by eighteen- to twenty-five-year-olds during the time of the pandemic. The dire need to shift how collegiate recovery functions and presents itself was made clear.

As the pandemic progressed, recovery meetings went online for months at a time. Students were stuck at the places they called home, some of which were not safe spaces for those in recovery. The difficulties in assisting collegiate recovery efforts only progressed along with the pandemic's spread. Leading, and participating in, recovery meetings on Zoom was a difficult adjustment to make. Students in recovery went from meeting face-to-face in a space that felt safe to speak about recovery to speaking about their

7. Executive Office of the President, "Declaring a National Emergency," 15337–38.

8. Richesson and Hoenig, "2020 National Survey on Drug Use and Health," 28.

9. Richesson et al., "2021 National Survey on Drug Use and Health," 32.

thoughts to a computer screen. Leaders of collegiate recovery were forced to limit their in-person interactions with students who were at risk. Nonetheless, recovery efforts, among every other aspect of human existence, must continue.

Collegiate Recovery After the Pandemic

It is the goal of collegiate recovery leaders to assist students who may be struggling even more with realigning after the pandemic due to substance use or misuse. Certain issues arose as a result of the pandemic for those in recovery including adapting to telehealth initiatives, the fear of the coronavirus driving up return-to-use rates, and compromised immune systems as a result of substance use and misuse.[10] The statistics mentioned in the previous sections of this chapter only confirm these fears from health professionals in the earliest days of the pandemic. With the goal of assisting students in recovery, CRP professionals are tasked to address and resolve these elevated issues moving forward out of the pandemic.

Not only did overall peer-support meeting attendance drop drastically coming out of lockdown, but the stigma of recovery seems to have returned as well. Whether this is due to the antisocial nature of the lockdown procedures or the result of shame and guilt for returning to use, the idea of moving forward remains difficult. A starting place for CRP professionals is to begin working on destigmatizing, modeling openness about being an individual in recovery, and assisting students in returning to face-to-face community.

The stigma behind substance use and recovery is debilitating. As members of the recovery community, students in recovery and CRP professionals know what it means to break stigma, and how to fail at breaking it too. There are countless studies on the psychological barriers that stigmas bring to a person who might be trying to better themselves. Keeping the substance use and recovery stigmas in place, or even outright ignoring them altogether,

10. Bebinger, "COVID-19 Outbreak Impacts," paras. 8–12.

leads to an increase in substance use and misuse by considerable factors. At minimum, if those misusing substances feel the stigma of getting proper treatment, the number of overdoses, and deaths, will continue to rise.[11]

So how do the barriers of stigma fall? Honesty and trust. These things are difficult to build and often take time to develop. A method many CRP leaders use is transparency "to the limits of institutional ability." There are certainly issues and facts that students should not know about staff or institutional operations, but being open and honest about one's own substance use and misuse history can be very beneficial for students. CRP professionals that are willing to disclose their own recovery, to the extent of their comfort level and established boundaries, can help tear down the walls of stigma.

Honesty and trust displayed by recovery staff may not be reciprocated, though it sometimes is. It is advised that staff members refrain from micromanaging or interfering with student peer support meetings. Nevertheless, promoting transparency can effectively reduce stigma within recovery spaces and throughout campuses. An institution that knows the goings-on of its recovery space is more likely to be invested in the CRP's current and future endeavors. It is likely that if the campus understands a CRP's recovery beliefs and efforts, the barriers to institutional assistance, both financial and otherwise, will begin to dissolve.[12] If CRP professionals attempt to hide their own recovery status from other departments or individuals across campus, they assist in reinforcing the stigmas that their students need deconstructed.

Whether resulting from substance use or not, CRPs likely have individuals in their recovery space that have compromised immune systems. The challenge in returning to "normal" after the pandemic was assisting these students with their return to campus and to recovery spaces. If such a student is present in a recovery community, the staff should provide them with any assistance or necessary freedoms they may deem necessary for them to feel

---

11. Volkow, "Stigma and the Toll of Addiction," 1290.

12. Yang et al., "Stigma and Substance Use Disorders," 384.

supported and included. If they choose to still wear a mask, staff can consider vocalizing the acceptance of masks in their space. If they need to continue using Zoom or other video methods to attend recovery meetings or other events, staff can designate a student or staff member to be their contact during those times. Being willing to work with, and for, uncomfortable or immunocompromised students is a vital effort for post-pandemic recovery.

Some students may react differently than others to these recovery initiatives moving forward from the pandemic, but these efforts will prove beneficial in the long run. CRP professionals should consider being open-minded about how their recovery community operates, markets, and intakes students. They can also consider contacting other CRPs or collegiate recovery leaders to communicate methods going forward. Finally, staff can access different training and educational resources that will provide them with the tools necessary to move forward in supporting students in recovery. Newer CRPs can begin by updating their language by going to the American Psychological Association (APA) website and learning recovery-minded language. There is also an extensive, though not exhaustive, list of recovery terminology at the back of this book.

At any stage of development, CRP programs and professionals should remember that the entire field is learning how to adapt and innovate recovery efforts. Students should be the greatest motivation moving forward in this unmapped territory. It is important to continually listen to students and their needs, as they might shift from program to program. Each student is different, and so is every recovery journey.

Chapter 2

Serving Students: What Does an Average Week Look Like?

Now that we have addressed the remaining pandemic, which is collegiate substance use, let us turn to more practical ways to serve students in recovery on college campuses. For this chapter, it will be helpful to address the heading initially, and then dive into each heading's content. This will give the reader an overview of the practical implementations for their recovery program, while still having the ability to navigate throughout the chapter.

The Goals of a CRP

The two most significant goals of CRPs to keep in mind are to provide an effective recovery community and to develop Recovery Capital (RC). The former will be the primary goal of a CRP in its relationship with students on campus, while the latter is a secondary, yet still extremely important, aspect of the program. We will explore ways to provide an effective recovery community below, but RC is a bit more complicated. RC is the availability and accumulation of resources one can access to support their own recovery or the recovery of others around them.[1] Developing an environment that prioritizes building RC is a "secondary" goal that is, in all senses, just as vital as providing an effective recovery community.

Recovery Capital is not built overnight. It is something that is not tangible, and one is not able to study its effects directly. What RC does provide is an increasingly strong recovery community that is exponential. Students who integrate into a CRP take away valuable knowledge and skills to share with other students, family members, and people in their community. This provides an excellent "spread" of recovery-mindedness that helps not just a local community, but the world we all live in.

The elements of RC are difficult to measure, as knowledge and skills are endless. There are, however, certain RC components that have been studied, and concluded to be quite essential no matter where one finds oneself in the recovery process. Proven beneficial RC elements include long-term recovery participation, the building of self-agency and problem recognition, an increase of social skills, a commitment to education or career goals, the establishment of personal recovery values, and the ability to have fun while sober.[2]

Possible Challenges/Things to Keep in Mind Moving Forward

The challenge one may face in determining their methodology week to week in a recovery program is that there is no set example that serves all institutions. Every CRP functions differently. A large R1 institution, for example, may have a different culture in its recovery space than that of a community college in a secluded area. This does not mean, however, that either is more important than the other. The two programs need only to realize that they will

1. Nash et al., "Exploring Recovery Capital Among Adolescents," 137.
2. Nash et al., "Exploring Recovery Capital Among Adolescents," 142.

function differently than each other, while keeping the well-being of their students at the forefront of their decision-making.

Keep this motivation in mind as this chapter is read. Students are the main priority. Methods that can be implemented will be discovered, which will allow for more RC moving forward. The mountain ahead may seem too steep, but the lasting effects of a program on its students in recovery are worth the climb. Keep pushing, maintaining students as the primary focus.

Weekly Meetings: The Vital Aspect

One way in which CRPs can serve their students, through both active recovery and RC-building, is by hosting and leading weekly recovery meetings. This is the most common method in CRPs, as it mimics the example outlined in the Alcoholics Anonymous *Big Book*. The reason this heading contains the word "vital" is due to the plethora of studies that uphold the effects of weekly peer-to-peer recovery groups.

Studies show that peer support groups, though not exhaustive in clinical studies, have proven to provide destigmatization efforts and long-term recovery support for people in active recovery.[3] Anyone who has been to both peer-support groups and clinical care can see the benefits, and negatives, of both functions. With weekly peer-support meetings, students in recovery can talk and learn together, while taking in others in recovery along the way.

Peer support groups can also help those who may not be in active recovery. Students who are not in active recovery can benefit from weekly recovery meetings as a good way to decompress and take a moment to be mindful of oneself during busy seasons. Both students in recovery and recovery allies should be encouraged to attend open CRP peer support meetings.

Support groups should be run by students, preferably student workers or interns. Undergraduates that have an increased interest in the recovery field, or who may be in social work,

---

3. Tracy and Wallace, "Benefits of Peer Support Groups," 152.

pastoral care, or other similar fields can take charge of peer support groups. Students in recovery often deeply resonate with their peers. Studies have also shown that leaders of peer support groups gain a better understanding of themselves and the recovery community as well.[4]

There are many commonly known peer support meetings that occur throughout the world weekly, so one does not need to worry about designing and building their weekly meetings from the ground level. This section will discuss the common, though certainly not exhaustive, types of weekly meetings that already have an immense network of resources, curriculum, and participant feedback to base a weekly meeting schedule on. These are good grounds to build on, but each CRP will be different.

The Twelve-Step Program: Alcoholics Anonymous

One of the most common peer support groups is Alcoholics Anonymous (AA). The *Big Book*, the main literature for AA, was first published in 1939 and was the first major implementation of a twelve-step program for alcoholism.[5] Although the twelve-step program, as well as the *Big Book* itself, has undergone tremendous amounts of revising and updating, it has remained a solid ground to build on in recovery from alcohol use disorder. The last significant update to the *Big Book* was in 2001, and since then recovery leaders have tended to shift away from the program in detail. The main themes and processes, however, are still used by many CRPs.

The twelve-step program, and specifically the *Big Book*, have obtained negative reviews in recent years for a few reasons. These issues rely on the fact that the two entities approach recovery from a Christian, mostly Caucasian, perspective that is not based on modern scientific methods. There have been voices from those in marginalized communities that have raised attention to the resulting harm that both the *Big Book* and AA have caused in speaking

---

4. Scannell, "Voices of Hope," 6.
5. Wilson and Smith, eds., *Alcoholics Anonymous*, xiii.

of the self, especially separating oneself from one's ego. Another critique of the two is that the twelve-step program is far less effective than the 75 percent success rate that the *Big Book* claims.[6] One study found that a closer estimate of actual success rate for the *Big Book* is somewhere around 5 to 8 percent.[7]

The last critique of the *Big Book*, and AA, has been its reliance on mainline Christianity, and the author biases that the book presents. Most of the steps are rooted in evangelical Christian values and morals that many people do not resonate with. This theme not only drives many people away from AA, but it also pulls many away from recovery in general due to the required belief in Christianity. When reading the *Big Book*, there is language about a "higher power," but for the original contributors to the book, that higher power was the American-Christian God.

While the *Big Book*, and the twelve steps in general, may cause certain issues among current students in recovery, the adaptability of the program can be beneficial for all CRPs. Using more inclusive language, while keeping in mind important aspects like the reliance on spirituality for recovery, can be more effective for a CRP operating in a diverse environment.[8] Even at religious colleges and universities, there will be students who do not believe in the God of Abraham or in Jesus Christ. Therefore, tailoring the language and methods of the twelve steps will likely be necessary to produce positive feedback.

While the customization of the twelve-step program is subjective, there are concrete ways to implement an alcohol recovery meeting from week to week. When there are fewer students in a particular semester, freedom exists to try new things. A book study, for example, can be done when there are fewer students. If there are more students, say twenty or more, then a peer-led curriculum is likely the best option for organizational purposes.

Weekly meetings will look a bit different, but the structure is generally three parts. It is beneficial to begin the meetings with

6. Wilson and Smith, eds., *Alcoholics Anonymous*, xx.

7. Glaser, "Irrationality of Alcoholics Anonymous," paras. 12–17.

8. Brown et al., "Developing the Spirituality in Recovery Framework," 11.

a general introduction to what the meeting is, and if students are comfortable, going around and saying their names.

After introductions have been completed, it is time for the meeting's contents. If the group is making its way through the twelve steps, talk about the current step the group is discussing. It can be helpful to mention its historical value from the 1930s, while also juxtaposing its current-day value. Talking about one's own experience with that step, if they are a person who has been in twelve-step recovery, can often resonate with the rest of the group. This is the moment in the meeting where questions about the discussed step are welcome and encouraged. At the end of this part of the meeting, students should have obtained a decent amount of RC regarding AA, and specifically, about the discussed step.

The final portion of the weekly meeting is the time to think about the near future. If the students are comfortable, the facilitator can ask them how their upcoming week is shaping up. What portions of the coming week are stressing them out? What portions are they looking forward to? The facilitator can also ask the students to share a moment that they know of coming up where they may be put in a situation where alcohol is present. This can often lead to a fruitful discussion about how the student can use their knowledge and skills acquired in a CRP in social situations. The student can then brainstorm their own plan to avoid alcohol at the event, and the group can encourage them with that plan.

There are other portions of these types of meetings that may be implemented, as well as parts that may be removed or shortened. What is most important is that the students lead the meeting. Their discussion and questions are the drive of their time together. CRP staff need to allow the students to manage the contents of discussion while steering the conversation towards encouragement and empathy. It is paramount to maintain an environment that is without judgment or condemnation.

There are many curricula for AA groups on the internet, as well as hundreds of books. This is a trial-and-error process. No CRP will be perfect. CRP professionals should keep their students in mind, and even ask them what they might find most helpful. If

AA is not a good fit for every student, there are a variety of other pathways to discover for student recovery.

SMART Recovery

Another solid option for weekly meetings is to run a SMART meeting. SMART is a nationwide organization that stands for Self-Management and Recovery Training.[9] The program is based on cognitive behavioral therapy (CBT), with the goal being for those in recovery to discover and train healthy coping skills for their lives. CBT has been researched as a positive treatment for many disorders, including SUDs and disordered eating.[10]

SMART meetings can be run with different types of curricula found online, and the organization provides training for facilitators of meetings. The capability to be trained in SMART meeting facilitation is the main draw of CRPs to SMART. Students can be trained in SMART and be allowed to plan and run meetings throughout any given semester. Something to note is that SMART training is not free and does take an estimated twenty total hours to complete.[11] The benefits of SMART training to students, however, are worth the time and cost.

SMART programs prioritize goal setting and taking applicable steps toward one's goals. There is often much time to analyze triggers, both past and forthcoming, to establish clear goals to reach beyond substance use. For this reason, many people in recovery enjoy SMART for its ability to apply the program during all points in a recovery journey. SMART participants also often explore new and different interests in an attempt to follow their goals, enriching the recovery experience for many involved.

---

9. Self-Management and Recovery Training (SMART), "About SMART Recovery," para. 1.

10. Murphy et al., "Cognitive Behavioral Therapy for Eating Disorders," 625.

11. Self-Management and Recovery Training (SMART), "Training Course Syllabus," para. 2.

One aspect of SMART that should be discussed is that it does not rely upon, or use any aspect of, spirituality in its recovery model. This is not inherently positive or negative, as it depends entirely on the individual participating. SMART is not "anti" spirituality, but it does not implement one's spirituality in the recovery process. This does not mean that someone in recovery cannot participate in SMART without spirituality. Spirituality and SMART can work concurrently to assist an individual in their recovery.

NAMI: Support for Student Mental Health

If a CRP and its leadership have the bandwidth, there remains the possibility to implement weekly meetings that do not necessarily have recovery as their main theme. One of those meetings is the National Alliance on Mental Illness (NAMI) meeting. This is a weekly, peer-led meeting that allows students to discuss their mental health and possible plans moving forward week to week to manage their mental well-being. NAMI, as an organization, has more than six hundred local affiliates and forty-nine state organizations.[12] Something important to note to students is that NAMI meetings are not a replacement for proper counseling services. CRPs must emphasize that proper mental health counseling is supported, and recommended, by the recovery space. NAMI meetings are merely a space to discuss one's mental health every week, not a place of treatment for mental health disorders.

NAMI meetings are structured similarly to other peer support meetings. Meetings begin with an introduction to the meeting, names, and, if students are comfortable, why they are attending the NAMI meeting. The main contents of the NAMI meeting are then discussed, using either the facilitator's own, or one of the many available, curricula. As with the AA meetings spoken of above, students should guide the conversation. NAMI is a time for students to decompress and discuss their current

---

12. National Alliance on Mental Illness (NAMI), "Who We Are," para. 5.

mental health struggles. It is imperative to allow them the room to lead the discussion.

NAMI is not an essential meeting for a CRP, especially if a CRP is limited in its leadership and schedule. It is, however, a concrete program that shows students the extent that the recovery community cares about health matters that often co-occur with addiction recovery. Hosting a NAMI meeting can benefit a CRP, even if only hosted monthly. CRP leaders can focus their ability to destigmatize and support mental health efforts without needing to host a weekly meeting.

Celebrate Recovery

Celebrate Recovery, or "CR," started in 1991 at the famous Saddleback Church in Lake Forest, California.[13] The ministry began to assist women and men who were struggling with chemical dependency and codependency issues within the large church. The first meeting contained forty-three women and men, and the ministry has grown to become a network of over 35,000 churches nationwide.[14]

There have been mixed reviews of CR in nonreligious communities, though CR and its effects have not been studied clinically. Most of the negative reviews of CR regard its functional purpose. The ministry's website states that the program exists as a Christ-centered, twelve-step recovery program for anyone dealing with hurt, hang-ups, and habits of any kind.[15] CR is a valuable recovery pathway for students who wish to attend a more Christian-centered recovery program. It should not be forced on any student. Personal spirituality certainly has a positive influence on an individual's recovery, but not every student who finds themselves in a

---

13. Celebrate Recovery, "How it Started," para. 2.
14. Celebrate Recovery, "How it Started," paras. 3–4.
15. Celebrate Recovery, "About," para. 1.

recovery space is Christian, and therefore should not be forced to participate in Christian recovery.[16]

Hosting Christian or other religious-based recovery meetings is not inherently negative. CRP leaders should evaluate their student population and make decisions accordingly. The last thing CRPs should be is another forced religion space, as many students who come to CRPs have been hurt by the church and may be weary of organized religion. Recovery staff members should be cautious to implement a CR weekly meeting without first discussing the desires of their student population. Again, students are the priority.

Meditations: Clearing the Mind on a Regular Basis

Another helpful weekly meeting is a guided meditation meeting. The structure of this type of meeting will certainly vary from CRP to CRP but is also more adaptable to different skills and schedules. Guided meditations can be held multiple times a week for fifteen to thirty minutes, or once a week for an hour, depending on the requests of students. The point of guided meditations is not to discuss anyone's progress or current recovery status, but instead to slow the mind and heartbeat to refocus on one's recovery and mindfulness.

As mentioned, the structure of guided meditations can fluctuate from program to program, or even from semester to semester within one program. The basic goal, however, remains the same. Slowing the body and mind, and focusing on mindfulness to achieve things like self-awareness, motivation, and discipline. There are many studies on the benefits of mindfulness in recovery, especially in intervening in SUDs and preventing return to use.[17]

CRP staff members can find guided meditations, or generally religious prayers, online and can lead students through them as a group, or individually, if requested. It is important to begin with a

16. Brown et al., "Developing the Spirituality in Recovery Framework," 11.

17. Priddy et al., "Meditation in the Treatment of Substance Use Disorders," 111.

time of focus. This can be done by guiding the student(s) through the closing of eyes, if comfortable, the taking of deep breaths, and the relaxing of shoulders, neck, back, etc. These steps, with the proper amount of time for each, will allow students to focus on being mindful for the duration of their meditation practice.

Just as the beginning is vital, so is the end of a meditative session. After the guided meditation has ended, it is important not to leave abruptly. It can be helpful to guide the students through a reorientation process. Some may have fallen asleep, which is perfectly fine and should not be met with punishment or judgment. The facilitator can simply tell them in a calm voice that the meditation is through, and that they may remain there or that they are free to leave if they wish. Again, the flow of these meetings is in the hands of participating students.

Meditations can be a simple, nondemanding way for CRPs to show students that they care about their holistic well-being. There are thousands of guided meditations and general spirituality prayers online that range in focus. It can be helpful to keep a running log of the ones that are used, so as to not use one too little or too often.

One-on-Ones: Helping Students Directly

Weekly peer-led meetings are one valuable aspect of recovery communities. Another way in which a CRP may assist its students is through one-on-one meetings. These are individual meetings between CRP staff and a CRP student. Having this option for students could prove beneficial to CRPs that have the bandwidth for such a method.

Some students within a CRP may not be "talkers" in group settings. This is perfectly normal and should be accepted with no issue. While these students may not participate in group settings vocally, they sometimes still need to be able to discuss issues with another person. Implementing a one-on-one environment can benefit these students. These quieter students may have issues that they want to discuss or may just want an individual guided meditation. It is CRP leadership's responsibility to provide students with the recovery support that they need.

Using a Google Calendar, Calendly, or other platforms can be an effective way to schedule individual meetings with students. QR codes or links can be posted on staff doors, in email signatures, and on marketing materials. This allows students to schedule one-on-one meetings quickly and efficiently, when needed. This type of meeting initiative can create safety and encouragement within a CRP and should be mentioned at the end of each meeting or event. Offering voluntary one-on-one services tells students that the staff is open to talking if they need or want to.

Something important to note about individual meetings is that they are not therapy sessions. Unless a CRP staff member is a licensed therapist, they are not trained to give mental health counseling. One-on-one meetings, in a recovery community, are intended to provide individualized recovery support. They can be a time to assess a student's RC and create tangible goals that students can work towards in recovery. Students will often approach their own conclusions and realizations in individual meetings. Simply having a non-clinical person to talk things out with is highly beneficial to students in recovery.

"Open Door" Policies

An "open door" policy connects with the previous section regarding one-on-one meetings. It also regulates healthy conversation and community-building within a recovery space. If a CRP is fortunate to have a recovery space with separate offices, keeping the door open when not busy is a great invitation for students to chat about anything from recovery and mental health to the local food spots and weather. Regardless of the topic, openness to conversation will prove positive to CRPs and will communicate to students that the staff members are approachable. Status signs can be posted outside of staff offices to tell students if staff are in a meeting, busy with something else, or free to talk. This is a helpful method of letting your students know that they can approach staff now or if they need to schedule for later.

Regardless of the institution, a CRP needs to welcome all students, regardless of race, color, religious beliefs, disability status, sexual orientation, or gender identity.[18] Inclusive CRPs should create an environment that has no tolerance for harassment of any kind in meetings or other events. A recovery community needs to establish a place of trust and belonging if meaningful recovery is ever to occur for students on campus. While many forces will attempt to alienate one or more of these marginalized groups, CRPs can create a sense of belonging for all of their students.

Maintaining Digital Community

Another vital aspect of a recovery community, especially in this technological age, is the implementation of a digital community. For this section, "Digital Community" may be defined as any virtual, and usually non-face-to-face, form of community. Especially after the pandemic, this aspect of CRPs is vital now more than ever. Students who may not feel comfortable showing up to in-person events still need community, as community plays a significant role in one's recovery process.[19]

There are many ways to implement and mold a digital community. Social media likely comes to the forefront of the mind when reading the term, but it is far greater than mere posts on an app. Although digital community may not be as effective or joyous as in-person community for some CRPs, it is a valuable alternative for students who cannot be physically present in recovery spaces.

---

18. McGeough et al., "LGBTQ Individuals Experiencing Substance Use-Related Problems," 229.

19. Boisvert et al., "Effectiveness of a Peer-Support Community," 217.

Using Social Media

As mentioned, social media is likely a primary aspect of digital community to most people. Although social media certainly has its limitations, using social media applications to relay important information and schedules to recovery students is quite important for any CRP. Social posts need not look professional, though a social media student worker is a beneficial hire if a CRP can justify one. Simply relaying when meetings are occurring, and where they are happening, is the minimum of CRP social media profiles. Taking advantage of commenting features can allow students to ask important event questions for clarification, which can be responded to by CRP staff relatively quickly.

Beyond times and locations of meetings and events, CRPs can use social media to highlight their students. It is important to get student permission before posting about them individually, especially if highlighting a recovery journey. Students who have excelled in their coursework or who have served in their local community may appreciate the public recognition. Posting a simple picture of them and sharing the CRP's pride towards the student(s) go a long way in developing a digital community.

GroupMe and Other Mass Communication Applications

Applications like GroupMe or WhatsApp are also important tools to use in any organization with a diverse population. There are certainly other programs like these to be used at the convenience of CRP staff and students, but these are two popular options. They are both able to be downloaded from the Apple app store, as well as the Android app store, so that most students can take advantage of the applications.

The basis of these applications is mass communication. Social media is helpful to relay information to those who may not be integrated into a CRP and to the public. Mass communications applications, however, are beneficial to the staff members and students who are part of a recovery community. Added simply through a phone number or username, students and staff are connected to one group message. This allows communication to reach staff and students directly on their smartphones. Some students may not check their emails regularly, so these applications may be more effective in reaching students quickly with important information.

CRPs can relay meetings and schedule information on these group messages, but they can also simply check in on their students as a whole at any given time. During school holidays or breaks such as summer or winter, CRP staff can check in on their students to see how they are doing. Having the convenience of these types of programs to communicate with an entire recovery community at one time is highly recommended for any CRP.

Texting and Direct Messaging

This aspect of digital community is a bit more subjective than the previous two. Texting and direct messaging (DMing) are great ways to check in on individual students privately. In the mass communication applications mentioned above, students who are struggling may not feel comfortable responding to everyone about their situation, which is where DMing and texting can be beneficial. CRP staff should allow the students to reach out directly first, to reduce pressure on students to answer their direct contact. Students may reach out through text or DM to discuss different aspects of their life, or simply to chat about a movie coming out soon. It is important that CRP staff implement proper boundaries, to protect work-life balance as well as the integrity of the professional relationship between staff and students.

Now that the basic centripetal functions of a CRP have been analyzed, this book will turn to the more centrifugal functions that can be modeled outside of a recovery space to drive recovery students into a CRP. These functions, like most mentioned here, are not exhaustive. They serve as a basis for CRP models to serve collegiate students to the utmost of the skill set available.

CRP Events: A Recovery-Minded Campus

One way in which CRPs can be external in function is by planning and hosting different recovery events around campus. These events can be a great way to spread awareness and destigmatize recovery throughout an institution and its student body. CRP events are difficult to suggest objectively, as they will depend on a multitude of factors including budget, marketing availability, student population, etc. One cost-effective CRP event to host is a sober tailgate at a sporting event on campus. Providing students an avenue to prepare for a sporting event without alcohol, or other substances, gives them the power to still have fun on campus without the triggers of the common college tailgate experience, which is heavily reliant on the use of alcohol.[20]

Collaborating with other departments on campus can mitigate event and marketing costs. This method will allow even the smallest CRPs to host events around campus on a somewhat regular basis. It also provides other departments on campus the opportunity to learn about, and invest in, the campus CRP. Cross-departmental knowledge is greatly beneficial to CRPs and students, both within the CRP and outside.

Orientations: A Freshman Introduction to CRPs

Another great way to get involved outside of a recovery space is to schedule events during freshman or transfer orientation times. Both setting up a table outside of student "hotspots" and hosting a breakout information session are concrete ways to spread recovery awareness to incoming students on campus. Giving new students access to contact the CRP will release one of the barriers that may stand between a CRP and students interested in recovery on campus.

Getting involved in an orientation program is often welcomed by new student programming departments. There is little cost, and, as long as collaboration is early enough, low impedance on

20. Oster-Aaland and Neighbors, "Impact of a Tailgating Policy," 281.

scheduling. CRPs can reach out to student recruitment or admissions offices to propose a CRP event during the next freshman or transfer student orientation. Letting incoming students know that there is a recovery space on their campus will decrease the stigma of recovery from the beginning of their time in higher education and promote a culture of inclusivity for years to come.

Recovery Housing

Many CRPs offer recovery housing for their students. Recovery housing is a designated residential space on campus for students in recovery. For some programs that lack a recovery center, recovery housing that includes a common space can also serve as a recovery center on campus. Some institutions are able to reserve an entire floor of a residence hall, while others can secure just a few rooms. Regardless of the number of beds available to a CRP, recovery housing is worthwhile to better support students who may be triggered by traditional dorms where substance use is commonplace. Even on "dry campuses," residence halls often find substances during room checks and encounter incidents with students who have been using substances. These traditional residence halls can jeopardize a student's recovery and often make students in recovery uncomfortable.[21]

CRPs can partner with residence hall directors to create a recovery housing program. Many institutions have an application process already in place for campus living, and CRPs can advocate for a question to be included that allows students to indicate an interest in recovery housing. These applications can then be sent to the CRP professional staff to review, engage those students in the CRP if they are not already, and select them for recovery housing. Another option is for CRPs to create their own application for recovery housing that they can share within their existing student community to then interview and place in available recovery dorms.

21. Bell et al., "'It Has Made College Possible for Me,'" 654.

Institutional Surveys/Polls: Learn What Your Students Need and Want

If a CRP is well-ingrained in its institution and receives a great deal of support from higher leadership, then utilizing institutional surveys or polls will likely help the program. Surveying the student body of an institution is the most direct method of figuring out what types of meetings and events are desired on campus. If a CRP is just getting established or has reached a stalling season, polling the students can lead to a necessary change in direction.

Possible Survey Methodology

Polling an entire campus of students is intimidating. There is an overload of information on official surveying and polling processes online, and in books, around the world. One word of advice on CRP polls: keep it simple. CRP staff members might not be trained in institutional survey implementation and analysis, so collaborating with the departments on campus that are trained in surveying will prove helpful.

It is useful to brainstorm the data that a specific program needs before creating the survey. Using metrics such as substance use history, gender orientation, religious beliefs, and others can allow a CRP to make structural shifts moving forward on campus. Asking for student religious beliefs, for example, can tell CRP staff the method and level of religiosity to use in their recovery programming. Asking for gender orientation can allow a CRP to implement certain safety measures for their students of different genders. These metrics, though vast, can assist CRP staff in creating programming that is better suited for their specific institution and student body.

If surveying is not a strength for a specific CRP's staff, they can reach out to a social work or science professor who uses surveying regularly. Many larger institutions will have specific survey and polling offices, which can assist a CRP in implementing campus-wide surveys. This method is good for those who are intimidated by campus surveys and will allow any CRP to have the opportunity to survey their student body.

How to Use Survey Results for Your CRP

The survey results are in, what's next? CRP staff are usually given a report of survey results, either in an Excel document from a Google Form survey or in another format given by the institution implementing the actual survey. Analyzing these results is what will assist CRP staff members in putting forth better-tailored programming. The basic use of survey results will vary across different programs, but the most significant insight is the needs of students.

Using the metrics given from a student survey, CRPs can create new programming, or shift existing programming, to assist in student recovery efforts more faithfully. For example, if survey results indicate that a significant number of students using substances identify as transgender, there may be an option to have an LGBTQ-specific meeting to help break up a barrier to recovery for those students. This example, though specific, is the general process for using and implementing survey results into a CRP.

Remember, also, that survey results can relay what a CRP is doing well also. Survey results might, for instance, speak to the amount of RC that the overall student body has, letting CRPs know that they have done well to educate and train students in the recovery field. It is important to understand how a CRP can shift using survey results, but it is equally important to understand what a program is doing well. This will not only validate the CRP's efforts, but also make sure that students are being served in the most effective and efficient way possible.

—————— Chapter 3 ——————

"Marketing" a CRP: Getting the Word Out

"Marketing" a CRP, which for this chapter means simply spreading word that a CRP exists on a specific campus, can be tricky. Nevertheless, some pointers for marketing a CRP will be discussed in this chapter. One thing to keep in mind when discovering the multitude of ways to market a CRP is that it is subjective per program. As mentioned before in previous sections, no CRP is set up or runs the same as any other. There are certainly similarities that likely outweigh the differences, but each campus is unique in its own way. Remembering this reality is what allows for a properly constructed marketing scheme for each CRP. This foundation will guide readers toward a tailored marketing strategy for their own campus.

Regardless of the institution, CRPs have the unique ability to provide recovery services to collegiate students for the sake of their overall well-being. Recognition of this privilege gives CRP staff a significant responsibility to discover how to best reach the student body as a whole. Each institution and its student body is unique. Remembering the opportunity that CRP staff have when analyzing a simplistic marketing strategy can allow for more determination and inspiration moving forward.

On-Campus

This chapter is divided into two categories of marketing a CRP. The first category is on-campus marketing. This process will come a bit naturally to most collegiate staff members, as there are no processes or pressures from outside of the institution they are housed in. Allocating on-campus resources to market a CRP comes as part of the job for CRP staff members. While there are multiple subcategories to observe, using on-campus resources, in general, is the recommended priority when marketing a CRP.

Student Organizations

Student organizations are one of the greatest avenues for assisting the marketing of a CRP on campus. Student organizations, and their focus, range from institution to institution. Regardless, dispersing responsibilities of marketing to different student organizations that may desire to be an integral part of a CRP is highly valuable. CRPs may also choose to begin their own student organization, such as a peer ally coalition, in an attempt to give students higher amounts of responsibility and leadership among their peers.

One of the most significant benefits of allocating student organizations for marketing purposes is that student organizations might have more bandwidth than that of CRP staff members. For example, there are times when colleges and universities hold student events during night hours, well past 5:00 PM. There may be no CRP staff member that can market the recovery community during this type of event, which has already been shown to reduce the risk of heavy alcohol use.[1] This is an example where a student organization can assist greatly. The student organization can take over at the nighttime event to run a table showcasing the recovery space. They can speak to the value of the space, and its necessity on campus. Not only does this give the CRP staff a chance to get home at a reasonable time, but it also allows the

1. Shotick and Galsky, "Impact of Late Night Programming," 20.

student body to hear from their peers about the nature of a recovery community, which is highly valuable to young adults.[2]

Several student organizations come to mind when considering the usefulness of their students to a CRP. The first is the Youth MOVE National (YMN). This organization, which advocates for uniting the voices of youth nationwide, has state and local chapters all over the country dedicated to assisting young adults in a variety of ways.[3] While some states do not have an official chapter established yet, there is constant work being done to establish chapters in all fifty US states.[4] Establishing an organization on-campus through YMN can allow students to receive additional peer mentoring and support. Partnering with such organizations can assist CRPs in a plethora of ways including additional hours of operation outside of a recovery space, an increase in destigmatization efforts across campus, and advocating for students' rights across campus and in local government.

Another student organization that can assist CRPs is a student government organization. These organizations are represented on most college campuses and serve students through advocacy, funding, and representational efforts. Partnering with student government organizations on campus can allow CRPs to allocate student leadership toward recovery efforts for the entire student body. At the same time, student governments can act as a mediator between institutional leaders and a CRP, which can benefit CRPs in the long run.

Regardless of the type of student organization a CRP may choose to partner with, their skills in marketing, strategizing, and implementation can certainly prove to be useful. Allowing students to market a CRP, even from within a student organization, is one of the most helpful implementations of student resources that any CRP can consider. The power of student voices backing a CRP should not be underestimated.

2. Moustafa, *Neural Aspects of Drug Addiction*, 260.

3. Youth MOVE National, "About Youth MOVE National," para. 1.

4. Youth MOVE National, "Chapter Services," para. 1.

Institutional Support

Marketing a CRP well relies heavily upon the institutional support that it receives. An institution's knowledge and support of a specific CRP can allow that CRP to allocate institutional resources in its marketing efforts. First and foremost, CRPs should prioritize regular and proper communication with higher leadership of their institution. Tell the president of the goings-on of the CRP that is starting, or that already exists, on their campus. If the highest leaders of an institution are unaware that a CRP exists on their campus, then effective marketing strategies will only run into increasingly difficult avenues.

Having the support of an institution also allows CRPs to take advantage of institutional marketing initiatives. Most colleges and universities have some type of social media accounts that have a following made up of current students, alumni, donors, and other institutional supporters. Being in good fellowship with the account owners and managers of these social accounts can allow for highlights of a CRP, or merely a post about the existence of a CRP on campus. This strategy is a simple way to market a CRP to already existing institutional followers.

Orientation Tables

Orientation is a time when an institution gains a significant number of new students, whether it is incoming freshmen, new international students, or transfer students. These incoming students, regardless of status, have a special opportunity to get involved in a variety of organizations and events across campus. If an institution has some type of tabling event or other organizational fairs, then it would be a beneficial marketing strategy to set up a table for a CRP at these types of events. It is relatively simple to reserve a spot at these events, so long as communication and scheduling are early enough for those organizing it.

The tabling itself is also relatively simple. Making flyers and other types of pamphlets to hand out to incoming students that highlight the CRP that exists on campus can give students the "in." Many incoming students do not know all of the organizations or offices that are there to serve them at their institution, so having a table set up at these types of events only benefits the students who are new to campus. Many students and their families are eager to learn about all the resources their new school has to offer.

When students approach a table for a CRP, staff should not be too forward or aggressive with their marketing strategy. Students are likely overwhelmed with the breadth of information already presented to them. CRPs would be wise to merely introduce what their space is set up for, who they serve, and a good way to contact the CRP staff. The interaction is more about connection than "selling" the program. This simple information, without pressuring students to come to meetings, is enough to let incoming students know that a CRP exists for them if they might need it during their time on campus.

Recovery Presentations

Recovery presentations educate the "public" about the current state of the addiction and recovery field. These can be done with as little, or as much, technicality as the presenter desires. It is important to know the audience of the presentation, so that the level of technicality may be determined appropriately. These presentations can be done for any group of people on campus, whether that is a student group, staff members of a specific department, or higher leadership members of the institution. Regardless of the audience and level of technicality, the goal is to educate those who are not a regular part of the CRP on up-to-date knowledge and methods of recovery.

While it would be helpful to discuss institution-specific recovery statistics and methods, it may not be necessary. It is common that most people on campus will likely have little awareness of the vast necessity for CRPs in college settings, seeing college substance and alcohol use as merely a social standard.[5] There is, however, a dire need to inform others about the statistics of nationwide addiction, especially in younger individuals. Giving these presentations or lectures allows CRP staff to further this education within their institution.

It is also possible to train students to give these presentations as peer educators. It is recommended that student presenters are chosen who understand the CRP more than the common visitor and that the student treats the presentation with sincerity and humility. Allocating students to give these presentations allows CRP staff to focus on other matters, and to remain present at the recovery space, as many recovery presentations will be given at different locations across campus.

Off Campus

On-campus marketing is certainly the primary marketing concern for most CRPs, but if a CRP finds itself well-known among its on-campus audience, it may be beneficial to market itself off-campus as well. Off-campus marketing can be intimidating, as the campus "bubble" must burst. There is often a significant difference in culture between a collegiate institution and its hometown.[6] With this difference in culture comes a difference in marketing strategy for CRPs in diverse cultural towns across the country.

Recovery Presentations

Like on-campus presentations, these off-campus recovery presentations are given in order to educate community members about the state of the addiction and recovery field. While the content of these presentations may be similar, whether given on or off campus, the delivery might be a bit unique. For example, giving a recovery presentation to a group of city government leaders will

5. Welsh et al., "Substance Use Among College Students," 117.
6. Chatterton, "Cultural Role of Universities in the Community," 177–79.

look different than giving one to a group of high schoolers in the city. The language and technicality of a presentation will shift depending on the audience off campus, but the goal is the same: to educate others on recovery.

There are many different places to schedule these types of presentations across any given city. Local religious institutions are a great place to begin. Most religious institutions have some type of smaller meeting (i.e., "small groups") that can benefit greatly from connection to outside groups.[7] Choosing which small groups to go to is the tricky part of presenting to local religious institutions. CRP staff need to be courteous and cautious about which institutions and groups within those institutions they choose to contact. Some religious institutions may not be so welcoming of clinical and technical presentations regarding addiction recovery, while others might desire education on the subject. While there is not an objective method of presenting in local religious institutions, if CRP staff members can find a group within one that desires recovery education, then partnering with such groups will lead to greater awareness and advocacy within the community.

Local nonprofits are another great audience for presentations across any city. Many nonprofits serve people who use substances, so educating the employees and volunteers of said nonprofits can be highly beneficial for the overall community. There could also arise opportunities to help serve these local nonprofits for CRP students who may be interested in volunteering. Partnering to provide presentations and services to nonprofits is mutually beneficial for both the organization and the CRP.

Local Religious Institutions

Partnering with religious institutions for the purpose of making marketing connections is up to the CRP and its staff. Religious institutions, however, can provide essential connections with students who may need to know that a CRP exists to serve them.

7. Bunton, "300 Years of Small Groups," 101.

Even in the smaller college towns, there are usually ministers at local religious institutions that are over the collegiate and/or young-adult populations at their specific institution. Connecting with these ministers can allow them to send her/his students to the CRP on campus if the student may desire to be connected. Partnering with these ministers also gives CRP staff the opportunity to visit with and educate the college students who attend that religious institution. CRP staff should be cautious not to overstep in any given college ministry and take care not to "take over" the college ministry from that minister.

Another helpful way local religious institutions can assist CRPs and their marketing initiatives is by hosting CRP meetings in their buildings, thus giving students an opportunity to engage in a spiritual community.[8] Some CRPs lack physical space for meetings on campus and could benefit from the available meeting space at a nearby religious institution. Not every religious institution will be open to hosting recovery meetings; but if one is, it will allow a window of marketing opportunity for the CRP in addition to a proper meeting space. Religious institutions often announce goings-on during their services. Depending on the institution, if a CRP meeting is occurring in their building, they might announce to the college students attending that this service is available to them if they desire it.

City Governments

Partnering with local government entities can also prove beneficial for CRPs and their student bodies. The methods of partnering with local governments are relatively subjective in terms of marketing, as it depends on the city that the CRP finds itself housed in. However, collaborating with local government officials can be a worthwhile endeavor for any CRP staff across the country.

City officials can assist CRPs by marketing their recovery residence to the members of the community that said information

8. Benz, *Recovery-Minded Church*, 135.

is relevant. According to a study done by the Society for Community Research, local governments are suggested to support, fund, educate, and train local recovery residences.[9] CRPs should, and can, take advantage of local government officials in order to reach other college students in the area that may not know of their program. Reaching all college students and other young adults within any given city is a goal that can be reached with the help of local government entities.

CRP staff can also advocate for their students and programming in local city government meetings and hearings, thus spreading awareness for the need of CRPs. Students may see this advocacy by CRP staff and be interested in certain CRP programming and initiatives. CRP staff should advocate for, and be the voice of, their student body across the city. This includes speaking out against local government laws and regulations that may be in place that hinder student recovery.[10]

Local Nonprofits

Using local nonprofits to market a CRP can be a fruitful endeavor as well. There may be CRP students or staff members that are already involved in a nonprofit in the area. If not, then connecting with these organizations can provide CRPs with an opportunity to reach more members of the community. Many college students take advantage of, or volunteer for, local nonprofits while on campus. More than 30 percent of college-aged students volunteer for local nonprofits regularly.[11] Allocating CRP students who volunteer, or participate in, local nonprofits can allow CRPs to spread awareness of recovery and of their space on campus.

These students who volunteer regularly at local nonprofits can take on the responsibility of gauging the educational needs of both the staff and other volunteers of the nonprofit. This gauging

9. Society for Community Research, "Role of Recovery Residences," 409–10.

10. Halvorson and Whitter, "Recovery-Oriented Systems of Care," 329.

11. Gazley et al., "Community-Based Student Learning," 1030.

will allow for possible presentations and/or training to take place at the nonprofit, thus further marketing the CRP and its services. This type of relationship with local nonprofits will allow CRPs to properly spread awareness and education about a variety of recovery efforts.

——————— Chapter 4 ———————

Intra-Institutional Addiction Recovery: Collaborating with Other Departments On Campus

COLLEGES AND UNIVERSITIES ARE systemic in nature, and a thriving CRP requires multidisciplinary support stemming from a variety of departments and resources on campus. To create strong relationships rooted throughout the university system, a CRP must find the delicate balance between exclusivity for students in recovery and inclusivity for recovery allies and recovery stakeholders. This chapter will discuss the threat of becoming a silo as well as strategies for building relationships with other departments on campus.

Operating a CRP Silo

One of the dangers of operating a CRP is becoming a silo on campus. Silos are departments or teams that work towards a mission or goal separate from collaborators and outside influences. Siloed CRPs develop for several reasons but can ultimately reinforce stigmatization and marginalization of students in recovery. Organizations operating as silos can hinder their own goals and threaten opportunities for collaboration among other departments that could serve as assets.[1] CRP staff may feel protective of their students, stigmatized by their institution's culture or values, or may simply feel misunderstood by other departments. Regardless of the underlying fears and beliefs, it is vital that CRP staff lean into their network to promote advocacy for collegiate recovery, continuity of student care, and holistic student success support.

Some universities are clothed in a culture of binge drinking that is pervasive across generations as alumni pass on legacies and traditions. Other institutions have religious affiliations that further nuance and stigmatize what it means to be in recovery. These are the institutions that tend to shield their CRP the most, often to avoid conflict and shelter their students from questions and criticism. However, these are also institutions that desperately need a voice for those struggling with substance misuse, addictive behaviors, and navigating early recovery.

To remain exclusive and to confine the recovery community to a small, secretive space on campus is to create a barrier to inclusive recovery culture on college campuses. CRPs with a desire to reduce otherness must make recovery spaces open and accessible not only to students but to faculty and staff. Shifting an institutional climate around addiction and recovery requires intervention at all levels of the university hierarchy. Faculty and staff that have never been to a recovery space or participated in a recovery meeting may be hesitant to advocate for CRPs as a resource on campus. However, personal experiences and relationships with CRPs can help faculty and staff create recovery networks throughout the institution.

Unapologetic recovery that is visible, consistent, and interwoven with campus-wide activities and initiatives reduces the marginalization of students in recovery. While CRP-specific events can build rapport among the collegiate recovery community and are valuable to CRP programming, engagement in cross-organizational

1. Bento et al., "Organizational Silos," 59–60.

activities and initiatives can increase awareness and comfortability with the CRP within the institution. CRP staff members must be intentional about forging collaborations with student life, student activities, athletics, campus recreation, and other departments to increase student engagement and recovery allyship.

The key to avoiding the CRP silo is intentional multidisciplinary relationship building. Every institution has recovery champions. Some 20.4 million Americans were diagnosed with an SUD in 2019.[2] Each of those individuals impacted many more loved ones around them. The likelihood that an upper-level administrator has been touched by addiction at some point in their lives is high. Through intentional relationship building, CRP staff can learn the stories of these recovery champions and share the mission of the collegiate recovery community. These individuals are stakeholders willing to advocate for a CRP despite working in another (sometimes seemingly unrelated) department.

How can CRP staff members build these relationships? Go to luncheons, professional development events, and open houses on campus. Invite leaders from other departments and student organizations to the CRP events calendar. Send out Christmas cards, valentines, and other notes from the collegiate recovery community to various offices on campus. Seek out professors interested in addiction recovery, build relationships with them, and ask who they know within the institution that also cares about this work.

Collaborating with Student Life, Campus Recreation, and Student Activities

Research indicates that students with a higher level of fear of missing out (FOMO) are more likely to engage in drinking alcohol and using illicit drugs.[3] To best support students in recovery, CRPs can collaborate across departments to provide student engagement opportunities rather than further isolating CRP students within a

2. Han and Piscopo, "2019 National Survey on Drug Use and Health," 3.

3. McKee et al., "Fear of Missing Out (FoMO) and Maladaptive Behavior," 8–14.

designated recovery space. Isolated students may turn to substance misuse in an attempt to cope with lack of connection. Well-connected CRPs can facilitate involvement in student activities, student networking, and substance-free fun on campus.

Student Life departments often provide education, outreach, and services that holistically support students. CRPs that actively partner with Student Life are able to plug their students into resources across campus that help them learn and grow as individuals, often in ways that support their recovery. Partnering with Student Life also sheds light on how CRPs can serve as resources for students on campus who may not yet be involved with the collegiate recovery community. Involvement with Student Life can expose students in recovery to additional student leadership opportunities as well as robust student programming.

Partnering with Campus Recreation promotes substance-free fun. Providing opportunities for students to connect through Campus Recreation affirms that substances are not necessary to form deep social bonds, and that recovery, along with holistically healthy living, can be rewarding and enjoyable. CRPs can get involved with intramural sports to increase teamwork among the community, challenge themselves mentally and physically on rock climbing walls, and can partner with Outdoor Adventures to enjoy wilderness retreats.

Student Activities departments generally house a plethora of student organizations, promote student events, and carry out campus traditions. Having a strong relationship with Student Activities allows CRP staff to stay in the loop regarding upcoming events and opportunities for their students. Getting involved with institutional tradition gives students in recovery a genuine sense of belonging on their campus and can increase school pride. CRP staff can co-host events with other student organizations to increase student engagement and promote awareness among various student groups on campus.

Collaborating with Title IX, Counseling, and Student Conduct Offices

Title IX offices, counseling centers, and student conduct officers are often on the front lines of identifying substance misuse and addictive behaviors. CRPs that wish to serve their institutions well and make the greatest systemic impact should strive to have deep, symbiotic relationships with each of these departments. Not only can these departments provide valuable referrals to CRPs, but CRPs can benefit greatly from having access to the resources provided by these offices.

Depending on the institution, CRPs are rarely clinical spaces, meaning they do not provide therapeutic intervention or clinical support. Therefore, the staff are mandated reporters for Title IX. Title IX offices protect students, faculty, and staff from discrimination on the basis of sex, including stalking, harassment, sexual assault, and interpersonal violence. Students can react fearfully when told that a Title IX report needs to be made after a vulnerable disclosure. Having a meaningful relationship with the Title IX office allows CRP staff to facilitate warm hand-offs for student care. This means that CRP staff can personally introduce the student to a trusted and close colleague in the Title IX office rather than offering a blind referral. Title IX cases often involve substance misuse, and survivors of sexual trauma are at an increased risk of misusing substances. Research indicates that over 3.5 million women abuse substances after being sexually assaulted.[4] CRPs can serve as a resource for Title IX offices as they work to support students on campus who may be struggling.

The counseling center often diagnoses students with SUDs or helps students gain insight regarding the severity of their addictive behaviors. Because counseling centers are confidential spaces, students are often more vulnerable and honest about their struggles with substances or other behaviors. Counselors can utilize their rapport with students to facilitate a warm hand-off to CRPs. On the other hand, peer support groups can provide space for

---

4. Kilpatrick et al., "Violent Assault and Substance Use in Women," 841.

students to share their deepest fears and struggles. CRP staff may identify students in need of higher-level mental health support. A strong relationship with the counseling center allows for CRP staff to better support students through the counseling center's intake process and creates opportunities for collaborative care if students wish for them to be included in their treatment.

Unfortunately for some students, the first time they realize they have a problem with substances or other addictive behaviors is when they are receiving consequences for misconduct. Student conduct officers often have difficult conversations with students as they enforce university policies. CRPs can offer student conduct officers resources and skills for talking about addiction and recovery with students they encounter. Additionally, student conduct offices can refer students to CRPs for recovery support to provide holistic student care rather than focusing solely on discipline.

Collaborating with Student Success Departments

CRPs aid in promoting student success for an often marginalized and stigmatized community of students. Student members of CRPs can include nontraditional college students that can benefit from additional support on campus. Being intricately connected to, and collaborating with, other departments on campus that support student success creates continuity of care for students in recovery that may need to utilize various support services.

Students in recovery can utilize departments of disability services to request accommodations when needed. This can be an intimidating process for students, and having CRP staff that is connected to the department and knowledgeable about the process can be greatly helpful. The mutual relationship also provides disability services offices with another valuable resource on campus for students.

Veteran Services is another crucial department for CRPs to partner with. It is not uncommon to have veterans in a collegiate recovery community. Access to peer support meetings and recovery support is also highly valuable to student veterans. Collaboration between CRPs and Veteran Services offers support for successful transitions and student experiences that foster connection for veterans.

Many CRPs offer a quiet lounge where students in recovery can study between classes. However, CRP staff can only provide so much academic support. To supplement their student success efforts, CRPs can collaborate with departments for academic success. Academic coaching and tutoring can benefit students in recovery as they pursue their degrees. An established relationship between academic success offices and CRPs can facilitate bolstered academic support for students in recovery.

Recovery housing can be an attractive aspect of CRPs. In order to provide dedicated space for students in recovery to live on campus, CRPs must partner with Residence Life. CRP staff can discuss needs for recovery housing with residence directors and even include questions regarding interest in recovery housing on institutional housing applications. Having a safe space to return home after juggling the many demands of college life can be instrumental for students' sustained recovery.

Collaborating with Spiritual Life Departments On Campus

There is no doubt that spirituality, in its most abstract sense, plays a significant part in the recovery process.[5] The twelve steps are built around the idea of a "higher power," which certainly can be the Christian God, but is not limited to just that. For this section, the sense of a higher power must be spoken of in a Christian sense. This section, however, is not limited to the Christian God just as the Twelve Steps are not limited to the God of the Bible.

There is an overwhelming number of religious higher educational institutions in the United States and Canada. According to the US National Center for Education Statistics, at least 862 higher

---

5. Brown et al., "Developing the Spirituality in Recovery Framework," 11.

education institutions in the country claim themselves to be religiously affiliated.[6] Undoubtedly, this number is not the whole picture, but rather a small looking glass into the number of institutions in the country that are likely to have spiritual departments embedded in campus life. In the Baptist world alone, over 830 institutions have an official Baptist Student Ministry on campus.[7]

There is no doubt that many college campuses in the country have some aspect of spiritual life on campus already. When planning a recovery program, it is essential to collaborate with those in leadership over campus spirituality. It is spirituality of the individual that is the strongest influence in one's recovery, and forming a CRP that is more coherent and functional requires collaboration with spirituality.

It is important to note that spirituality, in the sense discussed here, does not equate to Christianity or any denomination therein. Spirituality, in this sense, has to do with an individual's sensitivity or attachment to religious values. This definition comes with no certain religious bias, nor does it induce a certain belief system. Whether one is Christian, Islamic, Buddhist, or otherwise, spirituality in recovery is essential. It is vital to allow spirituality to inform the creation, or upholding, of a CRP.

One of the ways in which leaders of recovery initiatives can take advantage of their on-campus spiritual department(s) is through marketing, or outreach. In designing or implementing outreach for a CRP, the spiritual life department on campus can assist with the organization, funding, and workforce to implement getting the addiction-recovery word out.

Another way recovery initiatives can implement the assistance of spiritual life departments is through meeting spaces. Some CRPs are fortunate enough to have their own spaces on campus, though many are not. Most institutions with a spiritual department, however, have designated spaces, small or large, that can accommodate a recovery group throughout the weeks of classes. Merely the

6. National Center for Education Statistics, "Enrollment in Elementary, Secondary, and Degree-Granting Postsecondary Institutions," Table 303.90.

7. Oldham, "Baptist Collegiate Ministry," para. 2.

lending of an on-campus meeting space could be the difference in a CRP providing healthy recovery spaces for students.

The last practical way in which spiritual life departments can assist a CRP, though this is not a comprehensive listing, is through pastoral care. It is important to recognize the difference between addiction recovery, counseling, and providing pastoral care. Though the staff of an institution's spiritual department may perhaps have the proper training to provide immediate care for those in recovery who need someone to talk to, it is recommended that these staff members receive some type of addiction recovery training.

CRPs that have close ties to spiritual life departments are proven to be more effective in the long-term health of the student body. Relationships with these departments allow for greater marketing initiatives in tandem with the religious events happening on, and around, campus. There are often times, too, that students involved in spiritual life find it difficult to be open about their addictions. It is imperative that these two departments work together in order to diminish the stigma behind addiction and recovery.

With spiritual departments of colleges and universities joining hands with recovery initiatives on and off campus, there is adequate room for growth in recovery mindedness and a properly treated soil for a healthy student body. The necessity of spirituality in the recovery process is an undiluted truth that all leaders of addiction recovery need to recognize. The advantage of campuses with a spiritual life department is that students in recovery can be led spiritually in parallel to their recovery and vice versa, not in spite of it. The dichotomous attitude of colleges when it comes to spirituality and recovery proves only beneficial for students who are struggling with substance misuse or addictive behaviors on these campuses.

Chapter 5

Extra-Institutional Recovery: Working and Networking with Off-Campus Resources

Connecting with Other CRPs

WITH OVER 150 CRPs connected through the ARHE, it is evident that collegiate recovery is a growing field where professionals can navigate the job with help, eliminating the need to reach students alone. There are ample opportunities for recovery communities to network and collaborate. Despite the variation of programming and diverse student needs among unique institutions, CRPs can benefit from coming together for shared experiences, support, and continuing education for their staff as well as from providing co-hosted student events. There are several ways that CRPs can collaborate with others in the collegiate recovery field including conferences, virtual meetings, regional meetups, co-hosted events, tailgating at shared sporting events, and retreats.

Community is one of the most beneficial aspects of CRPs for students, according to a qualitative study.[1] A sense of belonging, shared experience, and peer support can help recovering students

1. Bell et al., "'It Has Made College Possible for Me,'" 654.

thrive on their campus. However, students are also making plans for their futures and are craving opportunities to create connections outside of their institutions. Community can be further amplified by creating shared experiences for students from various institutions to network, learn from one another, and support collegiate recovery. Students who take a special interest in advocacy and policy may also appreciate the opportunity to be involved in collegiate recovery at a macro level. These extra-institutional connections can serve students as they seek out graduate programs, career opportunities, and peer support groups as they move to new cities. The majority of CRP alumni feel that their CRP directly prepared them for the work environment as well as for post-graduation recovery.[2] To sustain this trend, CRPs should continue to provide networking opportunities for students in recovery.

Working in a CRP can be isolating within a larger higher education institution. CRPs often have a limited number of professional staff positions, and stigma on campuses can limit professional support systems. The unique demands of the job create a need for collaboration. Networking among CRP professionals is important for professional camaraderie and support, dissemination of wisdom, brainstorming new programming initiatives, and sharing resources. It can be validating to meet with other professionals facing similar challenges and who have shared goals and passions. Networking in the collegiate recovery field is also useful for the CRP to gain visibility; the more individuals who are aware that a CRP exists at a particular institution, the more likely that students in need will be connected to them.

A major opportunity to connect with many other CRP professionals and recovery advocates at once is to attend a conference. Conferences are highly useful for many reasons: continuing education units for staff with professional licenses, opportunities to network with other higher education professionals, workshops related to alcohol and other drugs (AOD) as well as recovery, and exposure to new resources. There are several local, state, and

2. Brown et al., "Alumni Characteristics of Collegiate Recovery Programs," 10.

national conferences that would be helpful for CRP staff to attend, depending on their goals. CRPs looking to connect with their own communities and partner with local organizations may benefit most from local conferences composed of interdisciplinary professionals and recovery advocates. CRPs interested in advocacy, policy, and state-specific resources may choose to spend their professional development budget on attending a state conference. CRPs hoping to meet a large number of other CRP staff members, learn more about national policies and resources, and connect with thousands of other higher education professionals, may choose to attend national conferences.

NASPA, the association for student affairs administrators in higher education, provides professional development, current research, and advocacy for student-facing professionals at over 1,200 institutions.[3] The annual NASPA Strategies Conference provides a plethora of workshops specifically addressing AOD prevention. This conference is frequented by collegiate recovery professionals as well as a variety of other prevention specialists that collaborate with CRP staff regularly. CRP staff members can not only learn about the latest trends in student alcohol and drug use as well as prevention, but can also acquire new skills, initiatives, and resources to further recovery efforts back on their campuses. There are often meetings scheduled among CRP professionals and advocates to network and share ideas directly related to recovery as well.

The annual ARHE conference is another opportunity for fellows in the collegiate recovery field to connect. This niche conference shares ethical considerations, standards of care, relevant research, and developments of collegiate recovery.[4] Hundreds of collegiate recovery professionals, students, and advocates gather each year to support one another and strengthen the field. The conference discusses diverse pathways of recovery, includes recovery

3. National Association of Student Personnel Administrators, "About NASPA," para. 1.

4. Association of Recovery in Higher Education, "2023 Conference," para. 1.

meetings for conference registrants to attend, and emphasizes the sustainability of the growing collegiate recovery field. Each year the conferences are typically held on university campuses with strong CRPs, allowing attendees to tour their recovery spaces and discuss programming that has been effective for their students.

The Higher Education Center for Alcohol and Drug Misuse Prevention and Recovery (HECAOD) is another resource that seeks to provide data-driven solutions to collegiate alcohol and drug misuse and recovery.[5] Each year they host an annual national meeting at The Ohio State University to connect prevention, early intervention, and recovery professionals to discuss the continuum of care. Collaboration among colleagues and the expansion of support networks allow for strengthened skill sets, interdisciplinary task forces, and education on evidence-based best practices.

Budgets for professional development may be limited, especially in newer CRPs or those that are lacking funded professional staff positions. Fortunately, there are several virtual resources as well as virtual meetings that occur weekly and monthly, providing collegiate recovery professionals with opportunities to network and gain knowledge and skills without the expense of travel and conference fees. ARHE hosts weekly staff chats for professionals to share experiences and strategies as well as learn from experts in the field, weekly all-recovery meetings for CRP staff members, and monthly harm reduction discussion groups. HECAOD provides free webinars and hosts "water cooler chats" for recovery professionals to network and learn. The *UReport,* sent weekly via email from HECAOD, is another helpful resource that includes the latest research summaries, open positions in the prevention and recovery field, and upcoming webinars and trainings.

For those that value in-person connection, regional meetups may be a good opportunity to network. Through connections made at conferences, utilization of the CRP directory on ARHE's website, and investigation of resources on nearby campuses, CRP staff members in a particular region can compile a list of potential

5. Higher Education Center for Alcohol and Drug Misuse Prevention and Recovery, "About," para. 2.

members of a regional community of recovery professionals. An email chain or group messaging app can be utilized to coordinate dates to meet up in a central location, as well as to facilitate regular communication and support between members. Parks, libraries, and campuses located centrally in the local region can make in-person connections accessible to all recovery professionals, students, and advocates who may be interested.

Multiple institutions may choose to co-host a shared event to bring their students and communities together. Universities may partner with their local community college for back-to-school bashes, or rival schools may co-host sober tailgates at sporting events. These shared events can expand recovering students' sober networks as well as provide a normative college experience, building RC while also increasing students' engagement with student life events. CRP staff members can plan for these events by looking ahead at the next semester's calendar, reaching out to other institutions to partner with, and marketing the event via social media and within the CRP for months in advance. For increased sustainability, partnered institutions can instill traditions in their CRP with annual events that may build momentum over time.

Retreats are another way to connect with other CRPs. Multiple CRPs can pool funds and plan co-hosted retreats. These retreats can be professional development opportunities for the CRP staff members and can be a community-building initiative for the CRP students. Bonfire recovery meetings, outdoor activities, educational workshops, guest speakers, and shared meals can all be enjoyed throughout a retreat. These retreats can become annual traditions within a region and can build relationships and awareness among local CRPs.

Connecting with Recovery High Schools

Recovery high schools are specifically designed to provide secondary education coupled with recovery support to students in abstinence-based recovery.[6] These schools give recovering students a normative high school experience while also helping them build a recovery foundation. Graduating students from recovery high schools often consider continued recovery support when applying to colleges or universities and may even seek out specific institutions to apply to their CRP. Over one-third of CRP alumni report that they would not have attended their institution had their CRP not been there.[7] By partnering with recovery high schools, CRPs can increase awareness of their programs to grow their communities. Partnering with recovery high schools also gives CRP students opportunities to mentor soon-to-be high school graduates.

Transitioning from a recovery high school to a CRP as a freshman in college is a natural graduation in the continuity of care for SUDs. First-year college students are at an increased risk for substance use, which creates a need for additional recovery support.[8] CRPs can support students in continuing to build on the RC established in secondary school and can provide a similar support system for recovering students. They can also serve as a protective factor as freshmen navigate the overwhelming first-year collegiate experience and develop peer groups on campus. Some CRPs are also able to provide scholarships, early admission, and priority registrations, thus reducing barriers to postsecondary education for students in recovery.

Recovery high school graduates make natural student leaders because they are equipped with strong recovery foundations and have experience with balancing recovery and schooling. In the context of peer support communities, having lived recovery experience makes these students inspiring additions to CRPs. These students are often candidates for student staff positions, peer group facilitators, and peer educators. Having student

---

6. Association of Recovery Schools, "What is a Recovery High School?," para. 2.

7. Brown et al., "Alumni Characteristics of Collegiate Recovery Programs," 10.

8. Skidmore et al., "Substance Use Among College Students," 746.

leaders can attract sober-curious students on campus and create organic peer mentorship.

One of the best ways to connect with recovery high schools is to create meaningful relationships with their admissions department, community relations department, or their counselors. Recovery high school staff members often attend the ARS annual conference that occurs in conjunction with the ARHE annual conference. This allows for convenient opportunities for CRP professionals and recovery high school staff members to connect. It can be helpful to invite stakeholders from recovery high schools to CRPs so that they can become familiar with the community space, programming, and CRP staff members. CRPs can also host "Open House" events for recovering high school seniors to attend, aiding in the seniors' search for the best institution and CRP to fit their academic goals and recovery needs.

Connecting Within the Local Community

Although institutions can create what may feel like an insulated bubble from the rest of the world, CRPs must create relationships within their local areas to bridge gaps in recovery services for students and the local community. These community relationships can raise recovery awareness, increase advocacy efforts, and decrease stigmatization of addiction and recovery. It can also increase access to much-needed funding and resources for CRP students and staff.

Although peer support meetings are a staple of most CRPs, varying student class schedules and availability can serve as a barrier to meeting attendance. Local communities often have a variety of meetings that can accommodate busy student schedules. CRPs can only provide so many types of meetings, and some students' needs may not be directly met. By partnering with local recovery chapters and meetings in the community, CRP professionals can help bridge the gap in recovery resources and diverse recovery pathways for their students. Not only is it useful for CRPs to have a calendar of local meetings and their details, but it can be helpful for CRP professionals to have direct relationships with attendees at those meetings, get an idea of the chapter culture, and develop familiarity with the location.

To foster the holistic well-being of students in recovery, it is paramount for CRPs to be connected to local community resources that can meet a variety of needs. Students may move on campus from hundreds or thousands of miles away and may lack familiarity with nearby resources. Local food pantries, low-cost healthcare, free or low-cost mental health services, temporary housing and shelters, and advocacy centers can be invaluable when students find themselves in need. Connecting with these community resources also provides volunteer opportunities for CRP students to be of service, thus fostering a mutually beneficial relationship between CRPs and local organizations.

Although CRPs are designed to support student recovery, return to use is possible. It is important to be connected to local SUD treatment programs in case students need a higher level of care. CRP staff who are familiar with various treatment options can provide insight and guidance to students who may be overwhelmed with their recent return to use or who may not have been to treatment before. It can be especially helpful for CRP professionals to have direct contacts in admissions at various treatment facilities for warm hand-offs when needed. Close relationships with treatment programs are also helpful to provide resources to individuals seeking higher education opportunities after treatment. Once an individual has completed treatment and built a foundation of recovery, CRPs can provide continuity of care for those choosing to pursue a degree.

Collaboration with Local Religious Institutions

Spirituality often serves as a catalyst for positive psychosocial changes in recovery.[9] Not all institutions have robust spiritual departments on campus, and thus relationships with local

---

9. Brown et al., "Developing the Spirituality in Recovery Framework," 10.

religious institutions nearby can be a beneficial resource for CRPs. The use of local religious institutions is advantageous for access to safe meeting spaces, spiritual guidance, and supportive communities. It is estimated that there are over 370 religious bodies, with over 356,000 congregations in the United States alone.[10] In Canada, the number of congregations of Christian orientation alone numbers in the thirty thousands.[11] Most college campuses in the world share a zip code with a plethora of religious institutions, therefore it must be considered that these institutions can assist a recovery effort on campus.

Some CRPs have access to meeting space(s) on campus for peer support groups. However, other institutions do not have a private space dedicated or available to CRPs, forcing recovering students to scramble to rent available classrooms or meet somewhere that lacks privacy. Church basements have historically been a meeting space for twelve-step meetings and other recovery groups. Religious institutions located near college campuses can provide cherished privacy and safety for recovery meetings.

Engaging in spiritual dialogue and having faith are significant aspects of recovery for many individuals. Conversing with diverse faith organizations within the local community allows CRPs to connect students with spiritual resources that align with their own beliefs. Navigating the acceptance of a higher power is nuanced and may be out of the scope of a CRP staff member. However, CRPs can still provide support by linking students with chaplains or local religious leaders as well as supportive faith communities.

10. Association of Statisticians of American Religious Bodies, "Press Release 2020," para. 2.

11. Hunt, *Handbook of Megachurches*, 270.

Chapter 6

Show Me the Money: How to Fund a CRP

Making a Case for a CRP

To ESTABLISH A CRP within an institution, one must first make a case and provide evidence for a need for such a resource on campus. When proposing the establishment of a CRP, it is important to have a calculated estimate of the cost and benefits of running these unique programs. Referencing campus-wide surveys and including evidence-based best practices will bolster the proposal. Statistics to consider include the number of students who disclose substance use, the number of students utilizing other institutional resources, the number of students who identify as being in recovery, and the number of students who withdraw from the institution due to reasons related to substance use. It can also be useful to put out a survey gauging student interest in a recovery program on campus and using those results to justify the proposal of a CRP.

The SAFE (Stop the Addiction Fatality Epidemic) Project is a nonprofit organization that provides advocacy and assistance for prevention, intervention, and recovery resources and initiatives. Their SAFE Campuses team assists those developing and maintaining CRPs.[1] SAFE Campuses has created resources for professionals who are building CRPs, and one that is particularly useful when considering funding is their CRP Business Case document. This document helps professionals calculate how many students their program could serve, the cost of student withdrawal for students who go without help at the institution, the seed funding needed to begin a CRP, and an estimate of how much the CRP would cost to maintain yearly.[2] This template is a great starting point for individuals interested in developing a CRP on their campus. Calculating these numbers can feel overwhelming, and some may not know where to start. The SAFE Campuses team also provides free assistance to walk through this guide.

How to Use Funds

Staffing

One of the key components of CRPs is professional staff members who facilitate programming and support students in recovery. It is ideal for a CRP to have at least one dedicated professional staff member, though most CRPs have two or more. Many full-time collegiate recovery staff positions require a master's degree and three to five years of related experience. This position requires a competitive salary as well as potential professional development funding to attract quality candidates.

Graduate student workers are another consideration when staffing CRPs. Working with graduate assistants can be less of a financial barrier than hiring additional full-time professional staff and can give graduate students valuable work experience. Graduate students can be incredibly valuable to assist in research, student mentoring, education and prevention efforts, and programming.

---

1. Stop the Addiction Fatality Epidemic (SAFE) Project, "SAFE Campuses," para. 1.

2. Stop the Addiction Fatality Epidemic (SAFE) Project, "Developing a Business Case."

These students typically work twenty hours or fewer per week, and their pay can range considerably depending on the institution.

Student workers are the heart of CRPs and often make up much of the staff. Because they are part-time and typically make close to minimum wage, CRPs can hire quite a few undergraduate students to help out in their space. Undergraduate student workers can help keep the space organized, facilitate peer support groups, assist in tabling and other outreach efforts, create content for social media, and many other tasks. Having student workers can allow the professional staff more time to focus on cross-collaboration with other institutional departments and community partnerships while ensuring that the inner workings of the CRP are cared for.

Creating a Space

While not all CRPs have their own physical space on campus, robust funding can assist programs in securing and developing a designated collegiate recovery center. The cost to renovate, furnish, and supply a recovery space can add up quickly. Many CRPs need couches or chairs, tables, desks, and other office furniture. Computers, a TV, and Wi-Fi can be additional costs to consider. For spaces that provide a community kitchen, CRPs will need to factor in the cost of a refrigerator, microwave, coffee station, and other kitchen appliances. While not necessary to begin a CRP, an established space on campus can solidify the program's existence within an institution and provide students in recovery with a safe space as well as a true sense of belonging.

Supplies

Another cost to consider for CRPs is the budget for supplies. Books, including twelve-step books, self-help books, and recovery workbooks, can be valuable resources to keep in the community space. Art supplies for experiential groups and student events can also be useful. Recovery chips are needed for celebrations of recovery and twelve-step meetings. Board games, card games, puzzles, and other activities for students to engage in as a community are beneficial to the recovery space as well. There will also be a need for general office supplies for staff members.

Promotional Items

Promotional items can be valuable in raising awareness of the CRP on campus. Tabling events happen throughout the year, and giving away promotional items is a popular draw for students to engage with the staff and learn more about collegiate recovery. Those students will then display the CRP's sticker on their laptop, wear their recovery T-shirt around campus, or drink from their CRP water bottle in class, providing additional marketing for the CRP. Promotional items can also create a sense of pride for CRP students and assist in efforts to destigmatize recovery on campus.

Feeding the CRC

Food is included in the monthly budget for most CRPs. If a recovery space has a refrigerator or pantry, the professional staff will need to keep the community kitchen stocked with soft drinks and snacks. Many student events on campus involve free food, which attracts higher student engagement. This is no different in recovery communities. CRPs will often need to budget for food when hosting student events. Coffee and tea are staples for many recovery spaces and should also be included in the budget for CRPs.

Retreats

Retreats, as discussed previously, can be valuable for the CRP. They do, however, come with a variety of expenses. Travel costs, groceries, lodging, guest speakers, activities, and supplies are all potential costs associated with facilitating a CRP retreat. However, CRPs can seek out donor funds specifically for retreats, organize retreat fundraisers, require students to pay partial costs or registration fees, and find other creative ways to gain funding if retreats are a desired activity among the students.

Scholarships

Some CRPs offer scholarships to students in recovery. The cycle of addiction can have a lasting impact on the financial well-being of individuals in recovery. These scholarships can make higher education available to students who may not have been able to otherwise afford it. While scholarship funds are usually limited, CRPs can create an application process for qualified students to at least have an opportunity for tuition assistance. CRPs can work with donors as well as their institution's financial aid office to create scholarship opportunities for their students.

Federal and State Funding

Several national government organizations have resources that CRPs can apply for. Substance Abuse and Mental Health Services Administration (SAMHSA) is one of these valuable resources. CRPs can apply for grants through SAMHSA on their website.[3] In the state of Texas alone, SAMHSA awarded a total of $102,714,355 in substance abuse funds in 2023.[4] Another valuable funding source is the National Institute on Drug Abuse (NIDA).[5] Recovery professionals can tap into these valuable resources by working with others experienced in grant writing. CRPs can partner with departments on campus, such as psychology or social work, to collaborate with seasoned grant writers to secure funding.

3. Substance Abuse and Mental Health Services Administration, "How to Apply," paras. 2–7.

4. Substance Abuse and Mental Health Services Administration, "Texas Summaries 2023," para. 3.

5. National Institute on Drug Abuse, "Grants & Funding," paras. 2–9.

Another financial resource for CRPs is state funds. A great starting place for many CRPs is their state health department. A specific state may have already been given funds for prevention and recovery initiatives.[6] Partnering with the state can also nurture a collaborative relationship between the CRP and larger systems to bolster advocacy efforts. Some CRPs already have relationships with their state health departments for naloxone and other valuable resources. Recovery professionals can build on those relationships to learn more about funding opportunities.

Institutional Funding

CRPs can tap into financial resources through their own institution as well. Most institutions have departments of advancement, donor relations, and foundation relations. These departments coordinate outreach efforts to foundations, connect with generous alumni, and connect donors to departments on campus. Having a relationship with departments engaged in funding efforts is beneficial for CRPs. It can be helpful to bring the departments' staff members into the recovery space, allow them to meet some of the community, and share the CRPs' mission with them. Having true investment from the institution's staff often facilitates being linked to the right donors who share a passion for recovery.

Alumni of the institution and the CRP are also resources for collegiate recovery communities. Alumni have deep emotional ties to the institution and/or the CRP, and often feel a desire to give back once they have graduated and secured successful careers. Having an alumni program can be a beneficial way to stay connected to the CRP's past graduates and can allow alumni to stay engaged with the CRP. This connection can foster donor relationships with alumni that would like to support students who have similar college experiences as their own.

Many institutions have a designated day for a mass fundraising event, often called "Giving Day" or "Day of Giving."

6. Independence Blue Cross Foundation and Association of Recovery in Higher Education, "Getting Started," 15.

The university puts in the legwork to market this day and raises awareness among potential donors including alumni, current students' friends and family, faculty, and staff. CRPs can piggyback on these efforts to raise funds for their students. Staff should be sure to mark their calendars for this day each year and connect with the appropriate department on campus to ensure their CRP is included as an option for donations.

Establishing the CRP's Presence

Presence on Campus

As mentioned in previous chapters, it is paramount that a CRP establishes a known presence within its institution. This visibility not only attracts students to the program but also attracts key stakeholders who may have an interest in financially supporting the CRP's efforts. Donors are drawn to programs that are actively engaged with students and that are making a visible impact on their campus. A CRP need not do anything extraordinary to attract stakeholders; rather, they should shine a light on the daily interactions and meaningful experiences of the students they serve. This authentic and organic presence will naturally attract passionate stakeholders who care for the recovery cause.

Presence Off Campus

Engaging off campus can be just as beneficial for CRPs as maintaining their presence on campus. Showing up in the community further destigmatizes recovery and raises awareness for the program and the students it supports. CRPs can maintain a presence off campus through service work with local nonprofit organizations, churches, and partnerships with departments of health and human services. These relationships can broaden a CRP's donor network by introducing CRPs to donors that support these partner organizations in the community.

Presence Online

In this modern technological age, a presence online cannot be over-emphasized. Not all donors will live locally or will be able to see the CRP live in action. This is one of the many reasons it can be beneficial for CRPs to utilize social media to amplify their presence and raise collegiate recovery awareness. An active social media presence reaches a larger audience than a website alone. Although an updated website can be a useful resource for individuals interested in learning more about a CRP, social media can be a more personal look into the culture and impact of a recovery community.

What does an active social media account look like? It doesn't have to be a perfectly curated grid of color-coordinated graphics and professional-grade marketing photos. In fact, that approach can hide the true culture of a CRP and can lack the authenticity that stakeholders may be interested in. Pictures of actual CRP students (who have consented to be shared on social media) can be the most effective draw to a social media following. Prospective stakeholders and students alike want to understand what CRPs do. CRP staff can increase intentionality by capturing a few pictures at every event, snapping candid shots throughout the week, and including pictures of student leaders and community members who would like a spotlight online.

These student photos give stakeholders a face to connect with the gift they have donated and can create a deeper meaning to their relationship with the CRP. Deepened relationships increase the likelihood that the stakeholder will continue to make regular gifts to the CRP, thus enabling the program to continue supporting recovery students. Simply documenting student support and sharing it online continues the cycle of financial endowment and can reduce the financial barriers that many CRPs face.

Updated websites are crucial for CRPs to share their mission, services offered, staff and student spotlights, resources, and upcoming events. Website links are a short and sweet way to share information about CRPs and can be utilized by fundraising departments on campus or CRP staff to quickly and efficiently educate others on who the CRP is and what they do. It can be helpful to embed short videos on the CRP's site touring their space, highlighting past events, or introducing students and staff. These videos can be shared via social media and email, and when interested individuals click on them, they will be directed straight to the CRP's website.

To best foster connection, a CRP's online presence should show more than it tells. When possible, photos and videos of the community should be used to demonstrate a CRP's mission and share about services offered rather than just listed information. Questions to consider when creating content to post online include "What does the CRP do?," "Why do they do it?," "What do they not do?," and "What impact do they have?" Capturing the stories and feelings of the collegiate recovery community can help enhance potential donors' understanding of the CRP's missions as well as emotionally appeal to those that may desire to support recovery initiatives.

Creating awareness through emotional appeal and organic content online is more likely to draw engagement from potential donors, thus increasing the likelihood of actually receiving a donation. Content can be repurposed for multiple uses, such as website content, social media posts, virtual newsletters, and follow-up emails. Repurposing content can strengthen the consistency of the CRP's messaging and cut down on some of the legwork of content creation for CRP staff.

Finding Prospective Donors

Donor audiences can include individuals in recovery, alumni of the institution or CRP, parents of students in recovery, and corporations with a special interest in recovery initiatives. CRPs can be connected to prospective donors through their institution, as discussed above, or through direct contact themselves. It is important to note that CRP staff should not supersede any institutional guidelines around cultivating donor relationships and should be sure to check with their department of development before proceeding.

Recovery champions are individuals in recovery or recovery advocates who contribute to prevention and recovery in many ways. This may be through promoting recovery-informed systems at an administrative level, mentoring and supporting others in recovery, or supporting prevention and recovery initiatives financially. The recovery field is well-connected, and working with recovery champions in any capacity can also provide networking opportunities to meet prospective donors.

Alumni often desire to give back to their alma mater once they have established themselves in successful careers. One study indicates that 68.2 percent of CRP alumni felt that their CRP prepared them for their professional environment, and 81.8 percent of them maintained contact with their former CRPs.[7] Students who feel strongly that their CRP played a significant role in their accomplishments post-graduation may be interested in paying it forward by contributing to a scholarship fund or donating in other ways.

Parents of students in recovery often express feelings of eternal gratitude to the CRP that helped support their child through his or her college career. These parents can feel called to invest in the center to ensure that other students and parents receive as much support as they did in their time of need. CRPs that include family programming often receive donations from parents and other family members that feel personally connected and invested in the CRP's mission and impact within its institution.

Nurturing Donor Relationships

CRPs are grateful for any financial gifts they receive. However, rather than receiving many small one-time gifts, a more effective strategy is to nurture donor relationships to increase the likelihood that they will continue to support students in recovery. Consistent connection and engagement with donors will

7. Brown et al., "Alumni Characteristics of Collegiate Recovery Programs," 10.

encourage gift renewals and help donors understand the impact of their donations. Personalized thank-you letters, invitations to CRP events, regular newsletters, and other forms of communication can deepen donor relationships and maintain interest in CRPs. Even when these outreach efforts do not result in new gifts, they can inspire donors to support the CRP in other valuable ways including volunteering, raising awareness, and sharing resources. Authentic and nurtured donor relationships increase funding potential for CRPs; well-funded CRPs result in better-supported students in recovery.

Conclusion

Where Do Collegiate Leaders
Go from Here?

THE GREATEST STEP ONE can take is to become a recovery champion. Maybe an institution is not equipped or funded or committed enough to start a CRP. Perhaps it has had a program in the past that disintegrated or was negatively received by the larger campus community. Even in these cases, collegiate professionals, key stakeholders, allies, and individuals in recovery can start by advocating for recovery-oriented systems within the institution.

A natural place to start is simply through the language used to describe students who use substances or students who are in recovery. Person-first language demonstrates the intentional focus on students as holistic individuals rather than oversimplifying them to stigmatized labels. Language is directly associated with feelings, and collegiate leaders have the power to associate recovery with hope, compassion, and resilience simply by being mindful of the language they use. Reviewing policies and documents used throughout the institution to modify any stigmatizing language is an attainable first step for higher education professionals to create change.

One of the most important changes an institution can make is in their language usage. Creating a cultural environment that is inclusive generates a sense of belonging and destigmatization for its students. Student well-being relies heavily upon their comfort within a CRP, so initiating proper language culture within a CRP will in turn create a more comfortable environment for all types of students within an institution.

Another opportunity for change is collaboration with the institution's student conduct department. Data from the previous years can be reviewed to understand the impact that substance use has had on the institution's student body. This data not only can be used to build a case for a CRP on campus but can also be used to assess how effective current student conduct policies have been. Recovery-informed professionals, like campus mental health counselors, can advocate for student conduct policies that connect students to resources rather than strictly punish students who have violated AOD policies on campus. This creates systemic compassion and policies that build RC for students struggling with substance use.

AOD education and prevention can often build a bridge to a future CRP. Prevention specialists play a similar role to collegiate recovery staff in that they also provide presentations to increase awareness on the impacts of substance use and interact with students who have a history of substance use. AOD professionals also organically introduce multiple pathways to recovery by utilizing harm reduction strategies to educate students on how to alter their relationship with substances. AOD prevention and education professionals sometimes take on the dual role of also starting an institution's CRP, and this pairing suits the needs of some campuses.

Above all other steps to take after reading this book, CRP staff, or ones wishing to implement a recovery space on their campus or in their community, need to practice flexibility and willingness to evolve or change. Recovery is one of those fields that constantly shifts in its language and its methodology. Becoming stonewalled and stuck in a certain way of doing things can become harmful for the students attending a recovery program. Academic institutions have a whole new student body every four to five years, so methodology will likely shift, even if slightly, every four to five years.

What to Do When Feeling Unsupported?

There often comes times when those interested in leading recovery efforts feel unsupported, or even alienated, on campus and throughout other aspects of their lives. It can become easy to give up and "throw in the towel," and those who push on are met with an uphill climb in helping their students who are struggling. Assessing a situation in which recovery leaders feel unsupported can lead to a shift in the methods of recovery for students, which in turn can give students the utmost care and support.

The first step in deciding to implement a CRP on campus is addressing the actual need for one in the community. Many cities have addiction recovery meetings already established, whether meeting in churches, schools, or other locations. There may also be organizations such as counseling centers or otherwise that already have peer-led recovery meetings accessible to all students. Some institutions have a higher immediate need for a CRP than others, depending on the resources that surround them. Assessing the need for a CRP when feeling unsupported can lead to the realization that a campus might already have initiatives in place for assisting students in their recovery.

If there are no initiatives in place for student recovery, then a case needs to be made to institutional leaders that a CRP is necessary for student well-being. Although this is covered in chapter six, CRP hopefuls will benefit from collecting institutional-specific data on substance use in order to make an evidence-based case for the need of a CRP. On paper, the greatest barrier is financial in nature, so take advantage of state and national funding if that is a gap needing to be bridged.

Perhaps a CRP already exists on a certain campus but is at a stalemate. A stalling CRP can feel unsupported. It is easy to look at dwindling numbers and feel discouraged. However, even if only one student is attending meetings, the CRP is "successful." CRPs measure success quite differently than many other departments within an institution. If a CRP feels like it needs to be "revamped," then a proper institutional survey may be helpful. Drafting questions regarding the state of substance use, mental health, and general wellness can lead to changes in methodology for a CRP. Surveys can also tell CRP staff what exactly needs to be shifted or changed within their programs according to their student responses.

A second option for CRPs that are stalling or ones that desire a shift is to take student interest and advocacy into account for programming and general methodology. Students are the heart of every CRP, and they have a variety of skills and insights to allocate for any CRP. Polling just the CRP students alone can lead to necessary shifts in CRP programming and event scheduling. CRP students are closer to the student body than CRP staff, so taking their advice and recommendations will allow for CRPs to make necessary changes and shifts in implementations that can lead to increased support to the overall student body on campus.

There is a sense of support when backed by numbers of individuals who resonate with the mission of the CRP. To gain this support, professionals must find recovery champions within the institution and community to share the importance of the recovery program. This can be done through simple connection with people. Sharing more about one's vision for a CRP, passion for recovery in higher education, and identifying the student need can often resonate with individuals and inspire them to share their own experience and connection to recovery. Given the prevalence of SUDs, it is highly likely that many colleagues and collegiate leaders have been impacted by their own use or that of a loved one. These personal experiences fuel passion to make a difference on their campus, and CRPs can be a tangible result of that desire.

Another way to increase support when feeling unsupported is to join the plethora of recovery networks and associations that exist in the world. Checking out associations like ARHE and other similar networks is a great way to find support in the recovery field across the country. ARHE holds a national conference yearly, so these connections are available in-person on a large scale as well as virtually on a more regular basis. Finding other recovery leaders can make any CRP staff member feel supported and understood in their work.

When feeling unsupported, it is likely that the institution has lost sight of the reason for the CRP. It is the responsibility of collegiate recovery professionals to continue building a case even once a CRP has been established. There are new staff, faculty, and students transitioning into the institution's community regularly, and it is important that they receive the same messaging on the importance of a CRP as those who preceded them. Continuing to build the case also creates opportunities for continued funding and re-evaluation of the allocation of resources at an institution. Once a CRP exists, the case builds itself—students are actively benefiting from its existence, and their stories are invaluable.

What Can Be Learned from Students in Recovery?

Students in recovery have a lot to teach others about life and the human condition. One significant moral factor that can be learned from these students is resiliency. Any person that goes through recovery, regardless of what they are recovering from, have been at a disadvantage throughout the entire process. While some have a better experience than others, all are attempting to better themselves while facing hardship. Learning how to fight uphill battles despite the circumstance is something that all people, and students, in recovery can teach others.

Along with resiliency comes courage. The common phrase is that "admitting is the first step to recovery." However, this is not the hardest part of recovery. Taking the steps to make amends with those we've harmed, as well as changing our social structures among countless other difficult measures taken during recovery, take an immense amount of courage. Taking note of how students in recovery speak of their past struggles, and accomplishments, can teach others many things about being courageous despite the barriers they may face.

A third aspect to learn from students in recovery, though certainly not the last, is a striving for honor. Students in recovery who attempt to make amends with those they have wronged are attempting to uphold their honor, whether they call it that or not. Restoring one's honor is not easy, and takes much courage and resilience, but it is a journey that is admirable and worthy of acknowledgment. We must all learn from those in recovery that honor, when lost, can certainly be restored again.

Appendix 1

List of Known Collegiate Recovery Programs (CRPs)

*Note: Data taken from the Association of Recovery in Higher Education (ARHE) with proper permission. An up-to-date list of known CRPs can be located at the following website: https://collegiaterecovery.org/crps-crcs/.

Institution	Street Address	City	State	Contact Email	Contact Phone
Allen University	1530 Harden Street/Chappellee Hall 308	Columbia	SC	wthompson@ allenuniversity.edu	(803) 376-5700
Appalachian State University	614 Howard Street/ASU Box 32130	Boone	NC	howardaf@ appstate.edu	(828) 262-3148
Arizona State University	4701 W. Thunderbird Rd.	Glendale	AZ	Jessica.Keene@ asu.edu	(480) 965-3759
Augsburg College	2211 Riverside Avenue OGC Suite 204	Minneapolis	MN	Jensens@ augsburg.edu	(612) 330-1170

Institution	Street Address	City	State	Contact Email	Contact Phone
Baylor University	One Bear Place #97197	Waco	TX	Kelsey_Austin@baylor.edu	(254) 710-7089
Berkshire Community College	1350 West Street	Pittsfield	MA	lmattila@ berkshirecc. edu	(413) 236-1609
Bingham University	PO Box 6000 - AB203	Binghamton	NY	kpeabody@ binghamton. edu	(607) 777-3640
Boston College	140 Commonwealth Avenue - Office of Residential Life	Chestnut Hill	MA	oxfordju@ bc.edu	(617) 522-6833
Boston University	930 Commonwealth Avenue/ Wellness & Prevention Services	Boston	MA	shv@bu.edu	(617) 358-0485
Bridge Valley Community & Technical College	2001 Union Carbide Drive	South Charleston	WV	carla.blankenbuehler@ bridgevalley. edu	(304) 205-6705
Brown University	One Prospect Street	Providence	RI	Lindsay_garcia@brown.edu	(401) 863-2536
Cabrini University	610 King of Prussia Road	Radnor	PA	jb3464@ cabrini.edu	(610) 812-1266
California University of Pennsylvania	250 University Avenue	California	PA	michaels_r@ calu.edu	(724) 938-4775
Cape Cod Community College	2240 Iyannough Road	W. Barnstable	MA	mweir@ capecod.edu	(774) 330-4550

Institution	Street Address	City	State	Contact Email	Contact Phone
Central Michigan University	220 W. Main Street - Suite 202	Midland	MI	jmiller@1016.org	(989) 774-1220
Cheyney University of Pennsylvania	1837 University Circle	Cheyney	PA	fgoode@cheyney.edu	(610) 399-2440
Coastal Carolina University	100 Chanticleer Drive/ Jackson Student Union B202	Conway	SC	tnardin@coastal.edu	(843) 349-2776
College of Charleston	66 George Street	Charleston	SC	marchantww@cofc.edu	(843) 953-6630
College of the Holy Cross	1 College Street	Worcester	MA	jlagrutta@holycross.edu	(508) 793-2302
Community College of Philadelphia	1700 Spring Garden Street	Philadelphia	PA	pscoles@ccp.edu	(610) 389-2096
Concord University	PO Box 1000/D-142	Athens	WV	afedele@concord.edu	(304) 394-5187
DePaul University - HPW	2250 N. Sheffield Avenue - Ste 302A	Chicago	IL	kturne40@depaul.edu	(773) 325-4550
East Carolina University	1000 E. 5th Street - SRC Room 208-B, MS 407	Greenville	NC	trotters19@ecu.edu	(252) 328-5172
Eastern Washington University	255 Martin Hall	Cheney	WA	mmcclung@ewu.edu	(509) 359-2366
Elon University	100 Campus Drive/Campus Box 2510	Elon	NC	ckelly26@elon.edu	(336) 278-5013

Institution	Street Address	City	State	Contact Email	Contact Phone
Emory University	1813 Druid Oaks NE	Atlanta	GA	epeller@emory.edu	(404) 727-0395
Fairfield University	1073 No. Benson Road - Dolan Hall/ Rm 14	Fairfield	CT	larnold@ fairfield.edu	(203) 254-2146
Fayetteville State University	1200 Murchison Road/ Counseling and Personal Development Center	Fayetteville	NC	dhall9@uncfsu.edu	(910) 672-2167
Ferris State University	1019 Campus Drive, Room 201	Big Rapids	MI	ScottWinkle@ ferris.edu	(231) 591-3614
Florida Atlantic University	610 SE 19th Street	Fort Lauderdale	FL	mpapania@fau.edu	(561) 297-1023
Florida International University	11200 SW 8th Street	Miami	FL	eparris@fiu.edu	(305) 348-4020
Georgia Institute of Technology	353 Ferst Drive NW - Suite 238	Atlanta	GA	steven.kontos@ studentlife. gatech.edu	(404) 894-2575
Georgia Southern University	Center for Addiction Recovery/PO Box 7988	Statesboro	GA	bfrazier@ georgiasouthern.edu	(912) 478-2288
Gonzaga University	502 E. Boone Avenue	Spokane	WA	herrington@ gonzaga.edu	(607) 793-7743
Green River College	12401 SE 320th Street	Auburn	WA	jking@greenriver.edu	(253) 333-6016

Institution	Street Address	City	State	Contact Email	Contact Phone
Hazelden Betty Ford Graduate School of Addiction Studies	1521 Pleasant Valley Road/ PO Box 11, CO9	Center City	MN	apeltier@ hazeldenbettyford.edu	(651) 213-4334
Holy Family University	9801 Franford Avenue	Philadelphia	PA	kcaulfield@ holyfamily.edu	(267) 341-4014
Illinois State University	120 Student Services Building	Normal	IL	jllaurs@ilstu. edu	(309) 438-2564
Indiana University - Bloomington	506 North Fess Avenue	Bloomington	IN	crcs@indiana. edu	(812) 856-3898
Indiana University-Purdue University Indianapolis	IUPUI Campus Center Suite 270, 420 University Blvd.	Indianapolis	IN	erictesk@iupui. edu	(317) 274-4745
Iowa State University	A37 Friley Hall/212 Beyer Court	Ames	IA	brianv1@ iastate.edu	(515) 294-1099
Jacksonville State University	700 Pelham Road North - 140 Daugette Hall	Jacksonville	AL	lmccauleyjr@ jsu.edu	(256) 782-5475
Kennesaw State University	1085 Canton Place NW Bldg. 6000/MD 6002	Kennesaw	GA	srathvon@ kennesaw.edu	(470) 578-7849
Kent State University	1500 Eastway Drive	Kent	OH	jschell@kent. edu	(330) 672-2487
Longwood University	201 High Street/ Upchurch University Center 309B	Farmville	VA	johnsonss@ longwood.edu	(434) 395-2146

Institution	Street Address	City	State	Contact Email	Contact Phone
Louisiana State University	16 Infirmary Lane Student Health Center - Room 173	Baton Rouge	LA	dbureau@lsu.edu	(225) 578-5384
Loyola Marymount University	1 LMU Drive, MS 8475	Los Angeles	CA	fpiumett@lmu.edu	(310) 338-1821
Marquette University	1102 W. Wisconsin Avenue - Ste 130	Milwaukee	WI	sara.e.smith@marquette.edu	(414) 288-5778
Metropolitan State University	700 East Seventh Street	Saint Paul	MN	maya.sullivan@metrostate.edu	(651) 793-1508
Michigan State University	556 E. Circle Drive/Rm 213 Student Services Bldg.	East Lansing	MI	Dawn.Kepler@hc.msu.edu	(517) 353-5564
Mid Michigan Community College	133 N. Saginaw Rd.	Midland	MI	Jmiller@1016.org	(248) 842-8746
Minneapolis Community and Technical College	1501 Hennepin Avenue South	Minneapolis	MN	jonathan.lofgren@minneapolis.edu	(612) 659-6468
Mississippi State University	84 Morgan Avenue	Mississippi State	MS	se126@saffairs.msstate.edu	(662) 325-7545
Monmouth University	400 Cedar Avenue - Office of Substance Awareness	West Long Branch	NJ	sschaad@monmouth.edu	(732) 263-5804
Montclair State University	1 Normal Avenue/Bohn Hall 4th Floor	Montclair	NJ	Schaferk@mail.montclair.edu	(973) 655-4155

Institution	Street Address	City	State	Contact Email	Contact Phone
Montgomery County Community College - Power Program	340 Dekalb Pike - PH210	Blue Bell	PA	nkang@mc3.edu	(484) 808-4223
Mott Community College	1401 E. Court Street	Flint	MI	dinah. schaller@mcc. edu	(810) 814-2308
North Carolina A&T State University	1601 East Market Street/ Murphy Hall/ Room 109	Greensboro	NC	vdbarnet@ncat. edu	(336) 334-7727
North Carolina Central University	1801 Fayette-ville Street	Durham	NC	jgrant31@nccu. edu	(919) 530-7646
North Carolina State University	2815 Cates Avenue/2101 Student Health Center	Raleigh	NC	jdfay@ncsu.edu	(919) 515-4186
Northampton Community College	3835 Green Pond Road	Bethlehem	PA	bmessina@ northampton. edu	(610) 861-5500
Northeast State Community College	2049 Rock Springs Rd	Kingsport	TN	dpwalker@ northeaststate. edu	(423) 943-4927
Norwalk Community College	188 Richards Avenue	Norwalk	CT	Wmendes@ norwalk.edu	
Ocean County College	1 College Drive	Toms River	NJ	khueth@ocean. edu	(732) 255-0386
Ohio University	Baker Universi-ty Center 321/1 Park Place	Athens	OH	addingto@ ohio.edu	(740) 593-4749

Institution	Street Address	City	State	Contact Email	Contact Phone
Oregon State University	108 Memorial Place Plageman Building - Room 117	Corvallis	OR	amy.frasieur@ oregonstate. edu	(541) 737-5041
Penn State University	106 Pasquerilla Spiritual Center	State College	PA	jxw411@psu. edu	(814) 404-4494
Pratt Institute	379 Dekalb Avenue	Brooklyn	NY	jmontoya@ pratt.edu	(718) 399-4545
Radford University	PO Box 7008	Radford	VA	cratcliff9@ radford.edu	(540) 831-5709
Ramapo College of New Jersey	505 Ramapo Valley Road	Mahwah	NJ	crosenkr@ ramapo.edu	(201) 684-7019
Renton Technical College	3000 NE 4th Street	Renton	WA	trable@rtc.edu	(206) 650-4910
Rowan University	201 Mullica Hill Road/ Wellness Center at Winans Hall	Glassboro	NJ	logan@rowan. edu	(856) 256-4333
Rutgers University - New Brunswick	17 Senior Street	New Brunswick	NJ	llaitman@ scarletmail. rutgers.edu	(848) 932-7884
Rutgers University - Newark	88 Linwood Avenue	Midland Park	NJ	barbaros. dinler@rutgers. edu	(973) 353-5805
Saint Joseph's University	5600 City Avenue/Champion Hall 231	Philadelphia	PA	tmoran@sju. edu	(610) 660-1149
Santa Clara University	500 El Camino Real/Wellness Center	Santa Clara	CA	kschumacher@ scu.edu	(408) 554-4448

Institution	Street Address	City	State	Contact Email	Contact Phone
Skagit Valley College	2405 E College Way	Mount Vernon	WA	Aaron.Kirk@skagit.edu	(360) 416-7849
Southeastern Louisiana University	SLU Box 10310	Hammond	LA	abladwin@selu.edu	(985) 549-3894
Southern Methodist University	6116 N. Central Expressway STE#205B	Dallas	TX	jmccutch@smu.edu	(214) 502-3222
Southern Oregon University	1250 Siskiyou Blvd.	Ashland	OR	damatoa@sou.edu	(541) 552-8464
Southwest Minnesota State University	1501 State Street	Marshall	MN	stacy.frost@smsu.edu	(507) 537-6483
Stanford University	581 Capistrano Way/Roger House	Stanford	CA	Clamb80@stanford.edu	(714) 605-1520
Syracuse University	Barnes Ctr at the Arch Hlth Prom - 150 Sims Drive	Syracuse	NY	banewton@syr.edu	(315) 443-0228
Temple University	1755 N. 13th Street - Student Center 201	Philadelphia	PA	TUWellness@temple.edu	(215) 204-8436
Texas A&M University	471 Houston Street	College Station	TX	sarahbethh@studentlife.tamu.edu	(979) 845-0280
Texas Christian University	TCU Box 297740	Fort Worth	TX	c.k.albritton@tcu.edu	(817) 257-7100
Texas Tech University	Box 41160/1309 Akron	Lubbock	TX	thomas.kimball@ttu.edu	

Institution	Street Address	City	State	Contact Email	Contact Phone
The College of New Jersey	Forcina Hall 308/PO Box 7718/2000 Pennington Road	Ewing	NJ	vaneck3@tcnj.edu	(609) 771-2134
The Ohio State University	113 W 12th Avenue/Baker Hall 095	Columbus	OH	hogan.180@osu.edu	(614) 292-0758
The University of Alabama	Box 870359	Tuscaloosa	AL	kelly.miller@ua.edu	(205) 348-2727
The University of Iowa	200 S. Capitol Street 19S0 UCC	Iowa City	IA	heidi-r-reyn-olds@uiowa.edu	(319) 335-7294
The University of North Carolina at Greensboro	Anna Gove Student Health Center 107 Gray Drive	Greensboro	NC	cakenne2@uncg.edu	(336) 334-4559
The University of Texas at Austin	2109 San Jacinto Blvd, E8000	Austin	TX	recovery@austin.utexas.edu	(512) 475-8352
The University of Texas at San Antonio	1 UTSA Circle - RWC1.808	San Antonio	TX	recovery@utsa.edu	(210) 458-8317
The University of Texas Permian Basin	4901 E. University Blvd.	Odessa	TX	carey_d@utpb.edu	(432) 552-3604
Thomas Jefferson University	321 Caley Ct.	King of Prussia	PA	yoonsuh.moh@jefferson.edu	(215) 951-2561
Tompkins Cortland Community College	170 North Street	Dryden	NY	afd004@tompkinscort-land.edu	(607) 279-2128
Towson University	8000 York Road	Towson	MD	zhitchens@towson.edu	(410) 704-2512

Institution	Street Address	City	State	Contact Email	Contact Phone
Tufts University	124 Professors Row	Medford	MA	ian.wong@tufts.edu	(617) 627-5495
University at Albany at SUNY	Health & Counseling Services - 1400 Washington Avenue	Albany	NY	llongo@albany.edu	(518) 956-8477
University of Akron	Polsky 415e	Akron	OH	jellis@uakron.edu	(216) 410-1861
University of Alabama at Birmingham	1714 9th Avenue, S. LRC 3rd Floor, Ste 380	Birmingham	AL	kpemslie@uab.edu	(205) 934-5816
University of Arkansas	525 N. Garland Avenue	Fayetteville	AR	magerard@uark.edu	(479) 575-2500
University of Birmingham	52 Pritchatts Road Edgbaston/Institute of Mental Health	Birmingham, ZAC B15 2TT		e.j.day@bham.ac.uk	(044) 121-3402
University of California - Berkeley	102 Sproul Hall, Barrow Lane	Berkeley	CA	beccagardner@berkeley.edu	(510) 664-4218
University of California at San Diego	9500 Gilman Dr. #0039	La Jolla	CA	collegiaterecovery@health.ucsd.edu	(858) 534-2158
University of California at Santa Barbara	Student Health Alcohol & Drug Program	Santa Barbara	CA	bryan-a@sa.ucsb.edu	(805) 893-7353
University of Central Florida	4098 Libra Drive - Bldg. 127 - Suite 309/PO Box 163333	Orlando	FL	crystal zavallo@ucf.edu	(407) 823-0776

Institution	Street Address	City	State	Contact Email	Contact Phone
University of Colorado at Boulder	119 UCB, 1900 Wardenburg Drive	Boulder	CO	christopher. lord@colorado. edu	(303) 492-9642
University of Colorado at Denver	900 Auraria Parkway	Denver	CO	recoverycom- munityinfo@ gmail.com	(303) 315-7270
University of Connecticut	626A Gilbert Rd., Wilson Hall A104	Storrs	CT	sandy.valen- tine@uconn. edu	(806) 486-8774
University of Delaware	231 S. College Avenue	Newark	DE	Jestok@udel. edu	(302) 831-3457
University of Den- ver - Health & Counseling Center	1931 S. York St.	Denver	CO	waltrina.de- frantz@du.edu	(303) 871-3699
University of Georgia	55 Carlton Street	Athens	GA	tvance@@uhs. uga.edu	(770) 542-0285
University of Houston	4161 Wheeler St. Rm 250 G	Houston	TX	jashifle@Cen- tral.UH.EDU	(713) 743-6143
Univer- sity of Mary Washington	1301 College Avenue	Fredericks- burg	VA	rtuttle@umw. edu	(540) 654-1660
University of Michigan - Univ Hlth Srvc Wolverine Wellness	207 Fletcher Street	Ann Arbor	MI	mattstat@med. umich.edu	(734) 763-1320
University of Minnesota - ROC	410 Church St. SE	Minneapolis	MN	Sanem006@ umn.edu	(612) 624-1940
University of Mississippi	980 Whirlpool Drive/So Camp Rec Ctr	University	MS	kloggins@ olemiss.edu	(662) 915-5055

Institution	Street Address	City	State	Contact Email	Contact Phone
University of Nebraska at Omaha	6001 Dodge Street HPER 102	Omaha	NE	unorecovery-community@ unomaha.edu	(402) 554-2409
University of Nevada at Reno	1664 N. Virginia Street MS083	Reno	NV	dfred@unr.edu	(775) 682-8514
University of New Mexico	MSC02 2220 Logan Hall 2100	Albuquerque	NM	mgoldberg@ unm.edu	(505) 277-0560
University of North Carolina at Charlotte	9201 University City Blvd. - Ctr for Wellness Promotion	Charlotte	NC	Kourso1@ uncc.edu	(704) 687-0175
University of North Carolina at Wilmington	601 South College Road/ Box 5992	Wilmington	NC	juskod@uncw. edu	(910) 962-4135
University of North Texas	1155 Union Circle #305008	Denton	TX	recovery@unt. edu	(940) 565-3177
University of North Texas at Dallas	1112 Dallas Drive	Denton	TX	constance. lacy@untdallas. edu	(972) 338-1381
University of Oregon	1590 East 13th Avenue	Eugene	OR	aforbes@ uoregon.edu	(541) 346-3227
University of Richmond	363 College Road/Well Being Center	Richmond	VA	hsadowsk@ richmond.edu	(804) 287-6368
University of South Carolina	1000 Blossom Street #301B	Columbia	SC	k.james@sc.edu	(803) 777-5781
University of Southern Maine	105 Payson Smith Hall/PO Box 9300	Portland	ME	christopher. corson@maine. edu	(207) 780-4678
University of Tampa	401 West Kennedy Blvd.	Tampa	FL	acarothers@ ut.edu	(813) 258-7363

Institution	Street Address	City	State	Contact Email	Contact Phone
University of Tennessee - Knoxville	1800 Volunteer Blvd. - Ste. 201	Knoxville	TN	smccall6@utk.edu	(865) 974-5881
University of Tennessee at Chattanooga	615 McCallie Avenue/Dept 1846	Chattanooga	TN	megan-mcknight@utc.edu	(423) 425-5265
University of Texas at El Paso	500 W. University/202 Union West	El Paso	TX	uteprecovery@utep.edu	(915) 747-8370
University of Texas Rio Grande Valley	1201 W. University Drive UC109	Edinburg	TX	christopher.albert@utrgv.edu	(956) 665-2574
University of the Science	600 South 43rd Street	Philadelphia	PA	sudi@usciences.edu	(215) 596-8877
University of Utah - College of Social Work	201 S. 1460 E. Room 330/ Ctr for Student Wellness/ Student Service Bldg	Salt Lake City	UT	wellness@sa.utah.edu	(801) 581-7776
University of Vermont	590 Main Street - Rm 112	Burlington	VT	amy.boyd.austin@uvm.edu	(802) 656-0236
University of Virginia	550 Brandon Avenue c/o Office of Health Promotion	Charlottesville	VA	jenniferhall@virginia.edu	(804) 586-7746
University of Windsor	401 Sunset Avenue	Windsor Ontario Canada N8S1A1	Canada	olabelle@uwindsor.ca	(519) 991-1926
University of Wisconsin at Madison	333 East Campus Mall - Rm 4413	Madison	WI	jenny.damask@wisc.edu	(608) 265-4901

Institution	Street Address	City	State	Contact Email	Contact Phone
Ursinus College	601 E. Main Street	Collegeville	PA	kbean@ ursinus.edu	(610) 409-3562
Vanderbilt University	2301 Vander-bilt Place	Nashville	TN	katherine.s.drotos@ vanderbilt.edu	
Villanova University	800 Lancaster Avenue	Villanova	PA	sean.dinan@ villanova.edu	(610) 519-4040
Virginia Commonwealth University Wellness Resource Center	815 South Cathedral Place, PO Box 842008	Richmond	VA	bannardtn@ vcu.edu	(804) 366-8027
Virginia Tech	600 Washington Street SW	Blacksburg	VA	kaitlinc@vt.edu	(540) 449-5277
Washington and Lee University	University Counseling, 204 W. Washington	Lexington	VA	kluder@wlu. edu	(540) 458-4590
Washington County Community College	1 College Drive	Calais	ME	bfarrar@wccc. me.edu	(207) 454-1000
Washington State University	1125 NE Washington St/ Health Promotion/PO Box 642302	Pullman	WA	maarhuis@ wsu.edu	(509) 335-8784
West Virginia State University	125 Sullivan Hall, East/PO Box 1000	Institute	WV	toledoke@ wvstateu.edu	(304) 766-3262
West Virginia University	628 Price Street	Morgantown	WV	olivia.pape@ mail.wvu.edu	(304) 293 2517
Wytheville Community College	1000 East Main Street	Wytheville	VA	mbryant@wcc. vccs.edu	(276) 223-4837

Appendix 2

Glossary of Recovery Terminology

*Note: The appropriate language in the field of addiction recovery is ever-evolving. All professionals and allies in the field have the responsibility of educating themselves and being intentional about using language that is destigmatizing, inclusive, and person-first.

Addict: A term used to self-identify as someone who has a substance use disorder or someone who engages in a behavioral addiction (NOTE: should not be used to describe someone else; person-first language is more recovery-friendly and destigmatizing).

Addiction: A disorder characterized by urge to engage in maladaptive behaviors despite consequences.

Alcoholic: A term used to self-identify as someone who has an alcohol use disorder (NOTE: should not be used to describe someone else; person-first language is more recovery-friendly and destigmatizing).

Alcoholics Anonymous (AA): A mutual aid fellowship that utilizes a twelve-step program to support abstinence-based recovery from alcoholism.

American Psychological Association (APA): A scientific, professional, and academic organization which represents the study of psychology.

Association of Recovery in Higher Education (ARHE): A United States-based organization which supports, connects, and provides resources for CRPs and those who are in collegiate recovery leadership.

Association of Recovery Schools (ARS): A nonprofit organization which establishes high schools geared towards assisting and educating teenagers on recovery processes and language.

Big Book: A book authored by Bill W., titled *Alcoholics Anonymous.* The basic text of AA.

Center for Disease Control (CDC): A United States government agency which seeks to protect human beings from all diseases, both known and unknown.

Clean: A term used to describe the absence of substances in one's system (NOTE: This term associates use with being "dirty" and abstinence as "clean/pure," which can be problematic. This term is used less frequently among recovery circles that welcome multiple pathways to recovery.)

Collegiate Recovery Program (CRP): Also known as a Collegiate Recovery Community (CRC); a college or university-provided program that provides a supportive community for those in recovery from substance use or misuse.

CRP Silo: A collegiate recovery program that is largely isolated within an institution, operating without collaboration or interdepartmental involvement on campus.

Department of Health and Human Services: A United States government agency whose primary goal is the health and well-being of the American people.

Fear of Missing Out (FOMO): The anxiety of being excluded from an event, friend group, experience, etc.

Higher Power: Something bigger than oneself; a key component to the twelve steps. Can be God, the universe, a twelve-step program, or anything else outside of oneself.

Naloxone: Drug used to treat opioid overdoses by blocking opiate receptors in the nervous system.

National Center for Education Statistics (NCES): A United States government agency that collects, analyzes, and releases information based on education in the US and other countries.

Overdose: A toxic amount of a substance.

Pandemic: A widespread outbreak of an infectious disease spanning an entire country or the entire world.

Recovery: The process of combatting an SUD or process addiction through treatment, coping skills, mutual aid support groups, abstinence, or other resources.

Recovery Ally: An individual that has not struggled with a substance use disorder or process addiction who supports and advocates for those in recovery from SUDs and process addictions.

Recovery Capital: The total resources an individual has to find and sustain recovery.

Recovery Champion: An individual who inspires others through sharing their own recovery journey or advocating for addiction recovery in the community.

Recovery Stakeholders: Individuals or organizations with key interests in addressing addiction recovery efforts.

Relapse: When an individual returns to use of substances or alcohol after a period of abstinence.

Return to Use: The recovery-friendly term to define what was previously known as a relapse; this is when an individual with an SUD starts using substances again.

SMART Recovery: Self-Management and Recovery Training; peer support groups supporting recovery through evidence-based techniques and skills.

Sober: Abstinent from drugs and alcohol.

Spirituality: The belief in something greater than oneself.

Stigma: The negative view of, or active discrimination against, a certain group of people based on characteristics of certain individuals in the group.

Substance Abuse and Mental Health Services Administration (SAMHSA): An organization within the United States Department of Health and Human Services that leads efforts to improve mental well-being of those with mental and substance disorders.

Substance Misuse: When someone is using substances for reasons that are unhealthy or opposite of their intended use.

Substance Use: Using a substance for its intended purpose, or in a casual/social manner.

Substance Use Disorder (SUD): A medical term given to those who are chemically dependent on substances. A more proper way to define someone than the stigmatized word *addict*.

Title IX: Civil law that prohibits sex-based discrimination in any schools; all federally funded schools have a Title IX department.

Twelve-Step Program: A recovery program guided by a set of principles, supporting individuals in abstinence-based recovery.

Withdrawal: Physiological and psychological symptoms experienced when an individual stops using a substance that they have become chemically dependent upon.

World Health Organization (WHO): A United Nations organization whose purpose is to promote health and to protect humanity from health issues of all types.

Bibliography

American College Health Association. "Reference Group Executive Summary Fall 2021." https://www.acha.org/ncha/acha-ncha_data/publications_and_reports/ncha/data/reports_acha-nchaiii.aspx.

Association for University and College Counseling Center Directors. "Annual Survey for Reporting Period July 1, 2021 through June 30, 2022." https://www.aucccd.org/assets/documents/Survey/2021-22%20Annual%20Survey%20Report%20Public%20FINAL.pdf.

Association of Recovery in Higher Education. "2023 Conference." https://collegiaterecovery.org/2023conference.

Association of Recovery Schools. "What is a Recovery High School?" https://recoveryschools.org/what-is-a-recovery-high-school.

Association of Statisticians of American Religious Bodies. "Press Release 2020." https://www.usreligioncensus.org/node/1641.

Bebinger, Martha. "COVID-19 Outbreak Impacts People in Addiction Recovery." https://www.npr.org/transcripts/820543018.

Bell, Nancy J., Kirti Kanitkar, Kimberly A. Kerksiek, Wendy Watson, Anindita Das, Erin Kostina-Ritchey, Matthew H. Russell, and Kitty Harris. "'It Has Made College Possible for Me': Feedback on the Impact of a University-Based Center for Students in Recovery." *Journal of American College Health* 57 (2009) 650–58.

Bento, Fabio, Marco Tagliabue, and Flora Lorenzo. "Organizational Silos: A Scoping Review Informed by a Behavioral Perspective on Systems and Networks." *Societies* 10 (2020) 56–83.

Benz, Jonathan. *The Recovery-Minded Church: Loving and Ministering to People with Addiction.* Downers Grove, IL: InterVarsity, 2016.

Boisvert, Rosemary A, Linda M Martin, Maria Grosek, and Anna June Clarie. "Effectiveness of a Peer-Support Community in Addiction Recovery: Participation as Intervention: Peer-Support Community." *Occupational Therapy International* 15 (2008) 205–20.

Brown, Austin M., Robert D. Ashford, Naomi Figley, Kayce Courson, Brenda Curtis, and Thomas Kimball. "Alumni Characteristics of Collegiate Recovery Programs: A National Survey." *Alcoholism Treatment Quarterly* 37 (2019) 149–62.

Brown, Austin M., Jessica M. McDaniel, Kelsey L. Austin, and Robert D. Ashford. "Developing the Spirituality in Recovery Framework: The Function of Spirituality in 12-Step Substance Use Disorder Recovery." *Journal of Humanistic Psychology* (August 2019) 1–15.

Bunton, Peter. "300 Years of Small Groups: The European Church from Luther to Wesley." *Christian Education Journal* 11 (2014) 88–106.

Case, Anne, and Angus Deaton. "The Great Divide: Education, Despair, and Death." *Annual Review of Economics* 14 (2022) 1–21.

Celebrate Recovery. "About." https://www.celebraterecovery.com/about.

———. "How it Started." https://www.celebraterecovery.com/about/history/our-history.

Centers for Disease Control and Prevention. "CDC Museum COVID-19 Timeline." https://www.cdc.gov/museum/timeline/covid19.html#.

Chatterton, Paul. "The Cultural Role of Universities in the Community: Revisiting the University-Community Debate." *Environment and Planning A: Economy and Space* 32 (2000) 165–81.

Executive Office of the President. "Declaring a National Emergency Concerning the Novel Coronavirus Disease (COVID-19) Outbreak." https://www.federalregister.gov/d/2020-05794.

Felson, Jacob, and Amy Adamczyk. "Online or In Person? Examining College Decisions to Reopen during the COVID-19 Pandemic in Fall 2020." *Socius* 7 (2021) 1–16.

Gandhi, Monica, Chris Beyrer, and Eric Goosby. "Masks Do More Than Protect Others During COVID-19: Reducing the Inoculum of SARS-CoV-2 to Protect the Wearer." *Journal of General Internal Medicine* 35 (2020) 3063–66.

Gazley, Beth, Laura Littlepage, and Teresa A. Bennett. "What About the Host Agency? Nonprofit Perspectives on Community-Based Student Learning and Volunteering." *Nonprofit and Voluntary Sector Quarterly* 41 (2012) 1029–50.

Glaser, Gabrielle. "The Irrationality of Alcoholics Anonymous." https://www.theatlantic.com/magazine/archive/2015/04/the-irrationality-of-alcoholics-anonymous/386255.

Halvorson, Angela, and Melanie Whitter. "Approaches to Recovery-Oriented Systems of Care at the State and Local Level: Three Case Studies." *Journal of Drug Addiction, Education, and Eradication* 9 (2013) 313–32.

Han, Beth, and Kathryn Piscopo. "Key Substance Use and Mental Health Indicators in the United States: Results from the 2019 National Survey on Drug Use and Health." https://www.samhsa.gov/data/.

Harris, Kitty S., Amanda K. Baker, Thomas G. Kimball, and Sterling T. Shumway. "Achieving Systems-Based Sustained Recovery: A Comprehensive Model for Collegiate Recovery Communities." *Journal of Groups in Addiction & Recovery* 2 (2008) 220–37.

Higher Education Center for Alcohol and Drug Misuse Prevention and Recovery. "About." https://hecaod.osu.edu/about.

Hunt, Stephen, *Handbook of Megachurches.* Brill Handbooks on Contemporary Religion 19. Leiden: Brill, 2019.

Independence Blue Cross Foundation, and Association of Recovery in Higher Education. "Getting Started: What You Need to Know about Building a Collegiate Recovery Program." https://www.ibxfoundation.org/pdfs/stop/collegiate-recovery-program-guide.pdf.

Kilpatrick, Dean G., Ron Acierno, Heidi S. Resnick, Benjamin E. Saunders, and Connie L. Best. "A 2-Year Longitudinal Analysis of the Relationships between Violent Assault and Substance Use in Women." *Journal of Consulting and Clinical Psychology* 65 (1997) 834–47.

McGeough, Briana L., Emera M. Greenwood, Nicole L. Cohen, and Angie R. Wootton. "Integrating SMART Recovery and Mental Health Services to Meet the Needs and Goals of LGBTQ Individuals Experiencing Substance Use-Related Problems." *Families in Society* 104 (2023) 222–33.

McKee, Paul C., Christopher J. Budnick, Kenneth S. Walters, and Imad Antonios. "College Student Fear of Missing Out (FoMO) and Maladaptive Behavior: Traditional Statistical Modeling and Predictive Analysis Using Machine Learning." *PLoS ONE* 17 (2022) 1–21.

Moustafa, Ahmed A. *Cognitive, Clinical, and Neural Aspects of Drug Addiction.* London: Academic, 2020.

Murphy, Rebecca, Suzanne Straebler, Zafra Cooper, and Christopher G. Fairburn. "Cognitive Behavioral Therapy for Eating Disorders." *Psychiatric Clinics of North America* 33 (2010) 611–27.

Nash, Angela J., Emily A. Hennessy, and Crystal Collier. "Exploring Recovery Capital Among Adolescents in an Alternative Peer Group." *Drug and Alcohol Dependence* 199 (2019) 136–43.

National Alliance on Mental Illness. "Who We Are." https://www.nami.org/about-nami/who-we-are.

National Association of Student Personnel Administrators. "About NASPA." https://naspa.org/about.

National Center for Education Statistics (NCES). "Enrollment in Elementary, Secondary, and Degree-Granting Postsecondary Institutions, by Level and Control of Institution, Enrollment Level, and Attendance Status and Sex of Student: Selected Years, Fall 1990 through Fall 2029." https://nces.ed.gov/programs/digest/d19/tables/dt19_105.20.asp.

National Institute on Drug Abuse. "Grants & Funding." https://nida.nih.gov/funding.

Oldham, Roger S. "Baptist Collegiate Ministry (BCM)." https://www.baptistpress.com/resource-library/sbc-life-articles/baptist-collegiate-ministry-bcm.

Oster-Aaland, Laura K., and Clayton Neighbors. "The Impact of a Tailgating Policy on Students' Drinking Behavior and Perceptions." *Journal of American College Health* 56 (2007) 281–84.

Pennelle, Olivia. "The History of Collegiate Recovery." https://collegiaterecovery. org/2019/12/20/the-history-of-collegiate-recovery.

Priddy, Sarah E., Matthew O. Howard, Adam W. Hanley, Michael R. Riquino, Katarina Friberg-Felsted, and Eric L. Garland. "Mindfulness Meditation in the Treatment of Substance Use Disorders and Preventing Future Relapse: Neurocognitive Mechanisms and Clinical Implications." *Substance Abuse and Rehabilitation* 9 (2018) 103–14.

Richesson, Douglas, and Jennifer M. Hoenig. "Key Substance Use and Mental Health Indicators in the United States: Results from the 2020 National Survey on Drug Use and Health." https://www.samhsa.gov/data/.

Richesson, Douglas, Iva Magas, Samantha Brown, and Jennifer M. Hoenig. "Key Substance Use and Mental Health Indicators in the United States: Results from the 2021 National Survey on Drug Use and Health." https:// www.samhsa.gov/data/.

Scannell, Christian. "Voices of Hope: Substance Use Peer Support in a System of Care." *Substance Abuse: Research and Treatment* 15 (2021) 1–7.

Self-Management and Recovery Training (SMART). "About SMART Recovery." https://www.smartrecovery.org/about-us/.

———. "Facilitator Training Course Syllabus & Outline." https://uploads. smartrecoverytraining.org/Library/Docs/Syllabus_GSF201.pdf.

Shotick, Joyce, and Alan Galsky. "Impact of Late Night Programming on Alcohol Use." *Journal of Alcohol and Drug Education* 57 (2013) 16–22.

Skidmore, Chloe R., Erin A. Kaufman, and Sheila E. Crowell. "Substance Use Among College Students." *Child and Adolescent Psychiatric Clinics of North America* 25 (2016) 735–53.

Society for Community Research. "The Role of Recovery Residences in Promoting Long-Term Addiction Recovery." *American Journal of Community Psychology* 52 (2013) 406–11.

Stop the Addiction Fatality Epidemic (SAFE) Project. "Developing a Business Case for Your Collegiate Recovery Initiative." https://docs.google.com/ document/d/1Em4jhEb-m4SL203SGTLS07YozJggXR9gWIDO8gKad YA/edit.

———. "SAFE Campuses." https://www.safeproject.us/campuses.

Substance Abuse and Mental Health Services Administration (SAMHSA). "How to Apply for a SAMHSA Grant." https://www.samhsa.gov/grants/ how-to-apply.

———. "Texas Summaries FY 2023." https://www.samhsa.gov/grants-awards-by-state/TX/2023.

Tracy, Kathlene, and Samantha Wallace. "Benefits of Peer Support Groups in the Treatment of Addiction." *Substance Abuse and Rehabilitation* 7 (2016) 143–54.

Volkow, Nora D. "Stigma and the Toll of Addiction." *New England Journal of Medicine* 382 (2020) 1289–90.

Welsh, Justine W., Yujia Shentu, and Dana B. Sarvey. "Substance Use Among College Students." *FOCUS* 17 (2019) 117–27.

Wilson, William G., and Robert Holbrook Smith, eds. *Alcoholics Anonymous: The Story of How Many Thousands of Men and Women Have Recovered from Alcoholism.* New York: Alcoholics Anonymous World Services, 1939.

Yang, Lawrence H., Liang Y. Wong, Margaux M. Grivel, and Deborah S. Hasin. "Stigma and Substance Use Disorders: An International Phenomenon." *Current Opinion in Psychiatry* 30 (2017) 378–88.

Youth MOVE National. "About Youth MOVE National." https://youthmovenational.org/about-us.

———. "Chapter Services." https://youthmovenational.org/chapter-services.